"High Blood Pressure Lowered Naturally"

(Atlanta, GA)

FC&A, a nearby Peachtree City, Georgia medical publisher, announced today the release of a new $3.99 research report for the general public, *"High Blood Pressure Lowered Naturally"*.

It reveals a startling new discovery at a world famous medical center: the reversal of high blood pressure without prescription drugs! A discovery unknown to most people.

What Your Doctor Doesn't Tell You

A recent U.S. Government survey revealed that most doctors don't tell their patients about the possible side effects of drugs they prescribe. Tell your doctor if you have any possible side effects given in this research report for high blood pressure drugs.

The Good Effects Of Lowering High Blood Pressure

You or those you love may take prescription drugs to lower blood pressure, relieve pain, reduce fluid buildup, regulate heartbeat or prevent strokes and heart attacks.

Dangerous Side Effects Of High Blood Pressure Drugs

Unfortunately, high blood pressure drugs can cause miserable side effects like headaches, poor appetite, upset stomach, dry mouth, diarrhea, stuffy nose, dizziness, tingling or numbness in the hands or feet.

Now Blood Pressure Can Be Lowered Without Drugs

Recently, a university study has proven that most cases of high blood pressure can be lowered without drugs. 85.3% of patients with high blood pressure were able to quit taking drugs.

Amazingly, their blood pressure remained lower than when they were on drugs. Cholesterol levels also dropped 26%. The doctor in charge said of this program, "You lose your tiredness. You feel much more active. You have a general feeling of well being."

How Did They Do It?

How did the hundreds of people in this study free themselves from the miserable side effects of drugs—drugs they thought they would have to take for the rest of their lives?

Why are medical doctors saying that the findings are "very exciting" and that many patients have "a new lease on life".

These questions are all answered in a new research report, *"High Blood Pressure Lowered Naturally"*. You can order it by returning this notice and $3.99 to the address below.

Easy To Read

Facts about lowering blood pressure without drugs are listed in 10 easy-to-understand sections. You'll learn about the latest research in nutrition. How the presence or absence of 4 minerals and 4 other nutrients in your food and water can dramatically change your blood pressure. How poisons in the environment can make blood pressure skyrocket! How relaxation training can help. Why blood pressure medicine is overprescribed.

FREE With Order

Order *"High Blood Pressure Lowered Naturally"* now and we will send you FREE, our newsletter, *Health News*.

You must cut out and return this notice with your order. Copies will not be accepted!

Order now! Tear out and return this notice with your name and address and a check for **$3.99** + $2.00 shipping and handling to our following address: FC&A, Dept. 4MZ-5, 103 Clover Green, Peachtree City, GA 30269.

Save! Return this notice with $7.98 + $2.00 for two books. (No extra shipping and handling charges.)

There's a no-time limit guarantee of satisfaction or your money back.

©FC&A, 1987.

"Prescription Drug Kills Doctor"

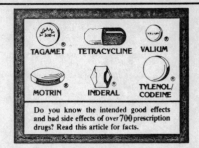

Do you know the intended good effects and bad side effects of over 700 prescription drugs? Read this article for facts.

(Atlanta, GA)

A local, Atlanta area medical doctor died from a freak drug reaction on a trip overseas. An infection he had didn't clear up after taking a drug; so he took a different drug, too. The two drugs reacted with each other and caused crystallization in his kidneys. He died with kidney failure a few days later.

What Your Doctor Doesn't Tell You About The Side Effects Of Prescription Drugs

This tragedy points to the fact that most doctors don't tell their patients about the side effects of the drugs they prescribe. This was revealed recently in a U.S. Government survey.

The reaction that killed the doctor and many other prescription drug side effects are clearly described in a new book, *"Prescription Drug Encyclopedia"* that you can order by writing to the address below.

The Good Effects Of Prescription Drugs

You take drugs prescribed by your doctor for their good effects, like relieving pain, fighting infection, birth control, aiding sleep, calming down, fighting coughs, colds or allergies, or lowering heartbeat and blood pressure.

Do You Have Any Of These Bad Side Effects

Prescription drugs can cause diarrhea, dizziness, dry mouth, depression, headache, upset stomach, constipation, stuffy nose, short breath, high blood pressure, fear and ringing sounds.

Do You Know The Answers To These Questions About Prescription Drugs?

When your busy doctor gives you a prescription, what do you, or even your doctor know about it? What's it for? Will you be allergic to it? What are its side effects and dangers? Will it affect other medicine you're taking?

One drug described on page 302 of the book can cause dangerous heart problems if you suddenly stop taking it. Page 40 warns that a drug you take routinely for shortness of breath can actually cause breathing difficulties! Yes, the very thing it's supposed to prevent.

Latest Facts On Each Drug

The book describes more than 780 of the most-often-used drugs. Facts are given in easy-to-understand words instead of hard-to-understand medical terms.

Easy To Read

Drugs are listed in alphabetical order for quick, dictionary-style finding. The book lists brand names, money-saving generic names, good effects, side effects, warnings and interactions with other drugs.

It explains drug categories. (For example: a drug may be called an "analgesic" . . . analgesic means "pain reliever").

Free With Order

Don't wait past the expiration date. Order this 30,000 word easy-to-understand book containing more than 780 drugs, edited by two pharmacists, and we will send you **FREE**, our newsletter, *Prescription Drug News*.

You must cut out and return this notice with your order. Copies will not be accepted!

Order *"Prescription Drug Encyclopedia"* now! Tear out and return this notice with your name and address and a check for $9.95 plus $2.00 shipping and handling to our following address: FC&A, Dept. DMZ-5 103 Clover Green, Peachtree City, GA 30269.

Save! Return this notice with **$19.90 + $2.00** for two books. (No extra shipping and handling charges.)

There's a no-time-limit guarantee of satisfaction or your money back. ©FC&A, 1987

Are You Taking Any of These Drugs? (Partial List of Drugs in Book)

Achromycin®	Cortisporin®	Erythrocin®	Larotid®	Ortho-Novum®	Synthroid®
Actifed®	Coumadin®	Erythromycin	Lasix®	Ovral®	Tagamet®
Aldactazide®	Dalmane®	Fiorinal®	Librax®	Parafon Forte®	Tetracycline
Aldomet®	Darvocet®	Haldol®	Librium®	Penicillin®	Thorazine®
Aldoril®	Darvon®	Hydergine®	Lidex®	Pen-Vee-K®	Thyroid
Amoxicillin	Demulen®	Hydrochloro-	Medrol®	Percodan®	Tigan®
Amoxil®	Dilantin®	thiazide®	Mellaril®	Phenaphen®	Tranxene®
Antivert®	Dimetapp®	Hydro Diuril®	Minocin®	Phenergan®	Triavil®
Apresoline®	Diuril®	Hygroton®	Motrin®	Premarin®	Tuss-Ornade®
Atarax®	Dyazide®	Inderal®	Naldecon®	Provera®	Tylenol/
Ativan®	E.E.S.®	Indocin®	Naprosyn®	Pyridium®	Codeine®
Bactrim®	Elavil®	Isordil®	Neosporin®	Septra®	Valium®
Bentyl®	Empirin	Keflex®	Nitrobid®	Ser-Ap-Es®	V-Cillin K®
Butazoladin®	Codeine®	Kenalog®	Nitroglycerin	Serax®	Vibramycin®
Catapres®	E-Mycin®	Kwell®	Nitrostat®	Sinequan®	Vistaril®
Compazine®	Enduron®	Lanoxin®	Orinase®	Sumycin®	

Please consult your physician before discontinuing any medication.

Vitamin and Mineral Encyclopedia

by Frank W. Cawood

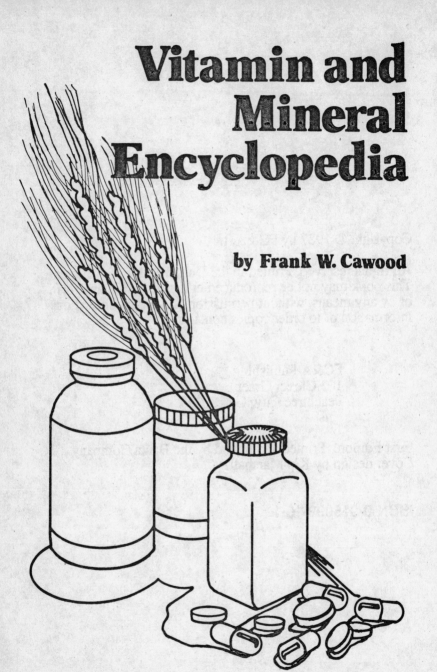

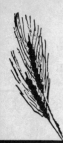

Acknowledgements

To my wife Gayle and my son Joseph, for their encouragement, constancy and support -- you have my earnest thanks.

Several other people gave their time and energy to help me write this book. Special thanks to:

. . . D. Carol Orleck,BSN, who researched and drafted part of the initial manuscript. Your patience and dedication is appreciated.

. . . Linda Sciullo for your typing and proofreading.

. . . Jan Ulery and Betty Whitfield, who strive for perfection in copy editing.

. . . Kip Marshall, who spent hours perfecting the cover, preparing the layout and paste up.

. . . Janice McCall Failes for coordinating production.

. . . all the supportive staff of FC&A, for their willingness to help in every way.

. . . But most of all, our thanks and praise is for our Lord and Saviour, who loves us, supports us and guides us.

Do you not know that your body is the temple - the very sanctuary - of the Holy Spirit Who lives within you, Whom you have received (as a Gift) from God? You are not your own, You were bought for a price   purchased with a preciousness and paid for, made His own. So then, honor God and bring glory to Him in your body.

-1 Corinthians 6:19 - 20 Amplified

TABLE OF CONTENTS

Introduction 15

Vitamins

Vitamin A (Retinol) 29
Vitamin B12 (Cobalamin) 35
Vitamin C (Ascorbic Acid) .39
Vitamin D (Calciferol) 47
Vitamin E (Alpha-tocopherol) 51
Vitamin K 57
Biotin 59
Choline 61
Folic Acid 65
Inositol 69
Niacin (B3) 71
Pantothenic Acid (B5) 77
Pyridoxine (B6) 81
Riboflavin (B2) 87
Thiamine (B1) 91

Minerals

Calcium 97
Chromium 101
Copper 103
Fluoride (Fluorine) 105
Iodine 109
Iron 111
Magnesium 115
Manganese 117
Phosphorus 119
Potassium 121
Selenium 123
Sodium 125
Zinc 127

An Amino Acid

Lysine 131

Other Books To Consult 133

Index 137

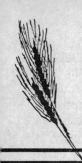

Introduction

Vitamin Pills ... Are They Good For You?

Vitamin pills ... are they good for you? The answer depends on whom you ask.

Dr. Alan Forbes of the United States Food and Drug Administration says that vitamins are widely available in good food and that there is no need for most of us to take vitamin pills.

Robert Rodale, the publisher of _Prevention_ magazine, says that taking extra vitamins, especially "natural" vitamins, is good insurance which can prevent or cure many diseases. His magazine is full of ads for vitamins, minerals and nutritional supplements for people who share his views.

Whom do you believe, the vitamin and health food advocates or the M.D.'s of the medical establishment? Even more importantly, why should you believe what I write in this book? Which side am I on? How can anyone know the truth in such confusion of contradictory opinions?

I am neither a medical doctor nor a vitamin advocate. I'm a concerned citizen who knows how to study scientific research and seeks to separate fact from fiction. This book is the prayerful result of much hard work to find out the truth about the benefits and hazards of taking vitamins and minerals.

As I did research, I decided to rely heavily on the

information in the U. S. Government book, _Recommended Dietary Allowances_, which gives a conservative opinion about how much of each vitamin and important mineral we need, plus many other widely accepted facts. I supplemented this information with a study of other authoritative reference books like _Facts and Comparisons_ and _Physicians Desk Reference._

These books became anchors as I examined many other books and popular articles about vitamins and minerals. If these other sources made reasonable, but unproven, statements, I attempted to verify them by going to original scientific articles for confirmation by controlled studies involving significant numbers of subjects. If I failed to get verification, I simply listed any unconfirmed benefits or side effects as just being claims or reports without expressing an opinion on whether or not they were true.

Because medical science is such a rapidly expanding field, new developments may have overtaken some of the information I have reported. Therefore, I ask that you consult carefully with your own physician before taking or discontinuing any vitamin or mineral supplement.

It can be dangerous to rely on self-treatment or home remedies and neglect proven medical treatments such as surgery in cases of cancer. A good physician is the best judge of what sort of medical treatment may be needed for certain diseases. It's good to choose a physician who has an interest in nutrition.

What Is, And What Is Not, Included In This Book

This book includes thirteen official vitamins and two near-vitamins. It also profiles thirteen minerals which have an important role in human nutrition, and one key amino acid, lysine. It doesn't include separate profiles for the many other amino acids which make up proteins.

Lysine has a special listing because it's often deficient in low protein diets from vegetable sources. Lysine also has unique properties which are being studied by many scientific researchers. Other amino acids also may have effects on the body which are not related to protein formation. As more scientific research on them is done, more amino acids may be included in future editions of this book.

What Are Vitamins And Minerals?

Vitamins are substances made by plants or animals that are needed by the body in relatively small amounts to help certain chemical reactions take place. They are found in some foods, and they are sometimes manufactured in the human body, usually by intestinal bacteria.

Like vitamins, some minerals are important in human nutrition. Minerals are not manufactured by living things. They exist in the rocks and soil around us, and the ones which are important in human nutrition usually can be found dissolved in many water supplies. Certain vitamins and minerals are essential for the growth, health and repair of the body as well as its routine functioning.

Enzymes are special molecules that usually are made by the body. They grab other molecules and put them together or break them apart. They help the body repair or defend itself, burn food as fuel or make its own building material.

Vitamins and minerals often link up with enzymes and activate them. They are like keys which help turn on many of the body's hundreds of enzyme-regulated engines. Vitamins and minerals also may have other roles in the body which are not related to enzymes.

Sources of Vitamins and Minerals

The best way to get the vitamins and minerals your body needs is to eat nutrient-rich foods. Fresh foods are generally the best sources of vitamins. Frozen foods are second best, and canned foods are a poor third. However, if you overcook your fresh food you may lose as many vitamins as are lost in canning food, except for carotene which is released by cooking. Light steaming is an excellent way of cooking which preserves more vitamins than other methods. Meat which is lightly broiled retains more vitamins than meat which is cooked in other ways.

The Benefits Of Taking Extra Vitamins And Minerals

There is much controversy over taking extra vitamins and minerals, but most medical doctors and nutritional authorities agree that some people can benefit from taking vitamin and mineral supplements in doses close to the Recommended Daily Dietary Allowance (RDA). Most authorities agree that the following people may benefit with improved physical or emotional health by taking extra vitamins and minerals:

- smokers
- surgery patients
- alcoholics
- pregnant women
- newborn infants
- people taking antibiotics
- runners and others who engage in heavy exercise or labor
- people, such as the poor and the elderly, who may have poor diets
- people on reducing diets

There is a lack of agreement among nutritionists about whether healthy people on a fairly well-balanced American diet can benefit from taking extra vitamins and minerals. Most nutritionists and medical doctors think that there is little or no benefit from taking extra vitamins and minerals if a person eats a well-balanced diet with foods from all four major nutritional groups. A minority of medical doctors and nutritionists think that the typical American diet is less than desirable, because much of our food loses vitamins when it's overcooked and overprocessed. They believe that modest vitamin and mineral supplementation is beneficial for the average American. An extreme position is taken by a small minority of people who maintain that taking large doses of vitamins and minerals can make a person "super healthy".

Research for this book strongly supports the middle position. There is evidence that most Americans can benefit by taking extra vitamin and mineral supplements in amounts which are close to the Recommended Daily Dietary Allowance or RDA. In my opinion, the only group of Americans who may not benefit from moderate vitamin and mineral supplementation are people, not in the above mentioned categories, who eat an exceptionally good diet. An exceptionally good diet is moderate in calories, alcohol, sugar, salt and fat. It is composed largely of whole-grain products, fresh fruits and fresh vegetables with moderate amounts of meat and dairy products. If people on such a nutritious diet also live in an area of the country where the water isn't "soft" they may get enough vitamins and minerals in their diet and drinking water for best health without taking supplements.

A key scientific paper by Enstrom and Pauling strongly supports the idea that taking a moderate amount of extra vitamins and minerals is best for overall health for most people. In this study of death rates among health-conscious elderly Californians, **the highest death rates occurred among those who took very high vitamin supplements.** The people with the lowest death rates and presumably the best health were those who took supplements in moderate amounts, not greatly exceeding the RDA's.

People who took supplements in moderate amounts generally had much lower death rates than people who took extremely high amounts of certain vitamins. The study specifically examined taking high doses of vitamin A, vitamin C and vitamin E. An increase in death rates was noted when people took more than several times the RDA for these vitamins. Unfortunately, the size of the study was too small to prove this conclusively for A & C, but it was big enough to prove this for E. This study casts doubt on the theories of those who advocate taking very large doses of vitamins or minerals for "super health."

This study also suggests, but doesn't prove, that people who take moderate vitamin supplements have lower death rates and better health than those who don't take any supplements.

The results of this study should not be used to rule out cautiously using large doses of certain vitamins to help correct certain conditions or enzyme-deficiency diseases like homocystinuria.

Vitamin And Mineral Supplements Can Cause Side Effects

Vitamin and mineral supplements can be good for most people, but this doesn't mean you should overdo a good thing. Vitamins and minerals can cause side effects, and large doses of some vitamins and minerals can cause serious side effects and even fatalities. It's usually safe to take vitamin and mineral supplements if you don't take more than the RDA, but you may do more harm than good if you take large doses.

The National Research Council's Food and Nutrition Board, which sets the U. S. Government RDA standards, defines a megadose as being ten times the RDA. When people take vitamins and minerals in megadoses they may run a risk of having serious side effects. Unfortunately, the government's definition of megadose is not a very good standard for determining whether or not a particular dose of a particular vitamin or mineral will be harmful. Some vitamins, like vitamin D, can be harmful when taken in doses above the RDA, but below the megadose level. On the other hand, some vitamins in the B complex are not reported to have serious side effects when taken at the megadose level.

In this book, I have tried to identify the dosage levels

for each vitamin and mineral where harmful effects have been reported to occur. Taking vitamins in doses up to these levels may not be a good idea, since it's difficult to determine exactly the dosages where bad effects outweigh good effects. There are sometimes indications of where this optimal level may be. For some vitamins and minerals, it may lie somewhere in the zone between the RDA and the level where harmful effects have been reported.

There are side effects and disadvantages associated with taking large doses of vitamins or minerals at levels which may not be high enough to be obviously harmful. Vitamins and minerals can have a general, stimulating effect on many bodily functions, including appetite. People sometimes become dependent upon vitamins. They may experience withdrawal effects such as irritability, upset stomach or depression when they stop taking large doses. Large doses of vitamins can be very expensive. Many medical doctors joke about people who take large doses of vitamins and say that they have the most expensive urine in the world, since the body quickly passes many water-soluble vitamins out of the body.

Vitamin pills can cause indigestion and even stomach ulcers, especially when taken with little or no liquid on an empty stomach. Vitamin C in the form of ascorbic acid and other acidic vitamins should always be taken after meals or with food or drink to dissolve and dilute the acid which comes in contact with the stomach.

Government Regulation Of Dosages

The U. S. Government is allowed by law to regulate the dosages of vitamins and minerals if there is proven harm to the public from taking large doses. The government has not used this power to stop the sales of large doses of the fat-soluble vitamins A, D, E & K, which can build up in the body and become harmful over time. It has regulated doses of folic acid, a rather harmless B vitamin when taken in doses a little bit above the RDA. Over-the-counter sales of folic acid are limited to 800 micrograms, because larger doses may interfere with tests to spot pernicious anemia and suppress some of its symptoms. This may not be good, because folic acid may help prevent heart disease in men and women and birth defects like spina bifida in the children of pregnant women. The optimal amount for preventing birth defects may be a little higher than 800 mcg. per day.

By the same reasoning, the government might limit sales of vitamin C, because taking large doses of vitamin C can interfere with tests for hidden blood in the stool, which can give early warning of intestinal disease. The reason the government has not done so may be the influence of a vitamin lobby that's supported by the many people who take large doses of vitamin C. Regulating doses of vitamin C may be politically more unpopular than regulating doses of folic acid.

Natural Versus Synthetic Vitamins

If you've ever gone into a health food store or a vitamin section of a drug store and read the labels on the vitamins, you've probably seen claims like "100% Natural", "Only Natural Fillers" or "Vitamin C With Rose Hips". Such advertising indicates that many people believe that vitamins from "natural" sources are better than vitamins from synthetic sources. This brings up the question of what is truly "natural".

The only vitamins and minerals that are truly, 100% natural are those which are found in food and drink. When people get vitamins free by choosing nutritious foods, they also get a bonus benefit of consuming the vitamins and minerals in a very natural state. Good foods provide vitamins and minerals which are bound to food, or at least mixed in with food, so that they come into the body unconcentrated. In many cases, these vitamins and minerals can help the body use the same foods in which they are found.

Any vitamins or minerals taken in pill form have been separated from food, and they come into the stomach in a concentrated mass. Vitamin and mineral pills can be irritating to the stomach and cause serious side effects, particularly if they are taken in large doses. Taking vitamins and minerals after meals may reduce stomach irritation.

Except for vitamin E, for most people it matters very little whether vitamins in pill form are from natural sources or synthetic sources. "A molecule is a molecule is a molecule" is an often quoted statement which indicates that the crystalline form of a vitamin from a natural source is identical to the same vitamin from a synthetic source.

People can buy vitamin C from a synthetic source at a very low price or pay many times as much for vitamin C which is extracted from a 100% natural source. In either case, the vitamin C will be identical in chemical structure no matter what the source was.

Naturally occurring vitamin C is sometimes found with substances called bioflavonoids which come from the pulp and the pith of citrus fruits. Bioflavonoids have beneficial vitamin-like properties, although they are not officially designated as vitamins. They seem to help strengthen the walls of capillaries or small blood vessels. Even though pure vitamin C from a natural source is indistinguishable from pure vitamin C from a synthetic source, a person might gain some benefit by buying a preparation of vitamin C which also included bioflavonoids. A person who did this might come a little closer to consuming vitamin C in the natural, fresh fruit state.

There may be undiscovered benefits to substances which are found with natural vitamins, that would not be present with synthetic vitamins. For example, there is an active form of vitamin E (d-alpha tocopherol) which is found naturally with other forms of vitamin E which have very little measured activity. It is theoretically possible that some of these other forms of vitamin E may have some as yet undiscovered benefits. A person can buy "natural" vitamin E found in mixed tocopherols at a considerably higher price than the same amount of vitamin E in the form of "natural" d-alpha tocopherol which may have been through more chemical processing.

Natural and synthetic forms of vitamin E are not identical. Vitamin E preparations designated, d-l-alpha tocopherol are a mixture of synthetic molecules which is not found in nature. The body may not always use or break down unfamiliar molecules as well as it does familiar molecules.

A very small percentage of people may be allergic to vitamins or to other substances found in vitamin pills. Some people can be allergic to natural substances found in vitamins derived from natural sources or to solvents used to process these "natural" vitamins. Others can be allergic to chemical residues which are found in vitamins that are synthesized or made by chemical reactions in a laboratory. Therefore, some people might have fewer side effects if they take vitamin pills from "natural" sources, but other people might have fewer problems if they take vitamin pills from synthetic sources.

To sum up my opinion on the debate about natural versus synthetic vitamins, natural is better than artificial, but truly natural means eating fresh, nutritious, vitamin-rich foods and not relying on pills to cover deficiencies from a poor diet.

The Meaning Of Terms Found On Vitamin Labels

An explanation of the following terms can help you decide how desirable it is to buy a particular product.

Buffered: A preparation which has been mixed with an ingredient which keeps it from becoming too acidic or too alkaline when it dissolves. This helps to prevent stomach irritation.

Time Release: Time release preparations have part or all of the ingredients coated with a substance which dissolves slowly, so that most of the contents are released into the intestine instead of the stomach. This helps to avoid stomach problems in people with sensitive stomachs, and it also helps to release the vitamin slowly into the body instead of releasing it all at once. The normal path of vitamins and minerals entering the body is through the stomach. It remains to be proven if bypassing the stomach and the bile duct just below it, which helps regulate digestion and control ph (acid-base balance), is always good.

Chelated: Condition of a mineral or other substance which is bound to another molecule. This helps the substance to be released slowly or sometimes to be carried into the bloodstream in its bound form. Organically bound minerals may be a little gentler on the body's digestive tract than pure minerals, but they may be more apt to pass through the digestive tract without entering the bloodstream than those which are not organically bound.

IU: International unit. This is a measure of the activity of a vitamin and not its weight or amount. IU's are usually used for fat-soluble vitamins which may be found in various forms of different activities.

RDA: RDA means Recommended Daily Dietary Allowance, a dosage level which has been determined by the government to be safe and adequate for human nutrition.

MG: Milligram or one-thousandth (1/1000) of a gram. This is the unit of weight which is most commonly used for describing the amount of a vitamin or mineral in a preparation.

MCG: Microgram or one-millionth of a gram (1/1,000,000). This is the unit of weight which is commonly used for trace elements and certain vitamins which are needed in very low dosage.

Fat Soluble: A term used to describe "oily" vitamins like vitamin E, vitamin D, vitamin K and vitamin A. These vitamins are digested along with fats, and they are generally stored in the body much longer than water-soluble vitamins.

Water Soluble: A term used to describe vitamins which will dissolve in water and which can be eliminated from the body fairly quickly if an overdose is taken. People who take large amounts of water-soluble vitamins often take them several times a day to maintain high concentrations in the body's tissues, because the body continually gets rid of the extra vitamins through the kidneys into the urine.

How To Understand The Following Descriptions For Vitamins And Minerals

Name: This section gives the common vitamin or mineral name in bold face type, and alternate forms or spellings.

What It Does: This section describes the medically accepted functions of the vitamin or mineral.

Food Sources: This section tells how you can get this vitamin or mineral "free" just by being selective when you're purchasing your foods. The best sources are listed first.

How Long It Stays In Your Body: This section tells how long a vitamin or mineral stays in your body before it's used up or passed out with body wastes. Some vitamins and minerals can be stored in the body for a long time. Others may pass through the body rapidly and need to be replaced often.

Deficiency Diseases And Symptoms: This section discusses the medically proven effects when adequate amounts of the vitamin or mineral are not found in the diet, or when the vitamin or mineral is not absorbed properly into the body.

What Reduces, Destroys Or Increases It: This section lists many things such as methods of food processing and preparation, alcohol, prescription drugs, exercise, other vitamins or minerals or certain medical conditions that can destroy, reduce or increase the level or the activity of a vitamin or mineral.

Recommended Daily Dietary Allowance (RDA): This section lists the U.S. Government Food and Nutrition Board's official standard, the Recommended Daily

Dietary Allowance, which is the amount that they think best for overall health. This section also reports the government's "estimated safe and adequate daily dietary intakes" for those vitamins or minerals which do not yet have established RDA's. Most of the figures given for minerals are estimates rather than official RDA's. RDA's are reported in milligrams (mg.) = 1/1000 of a gram, micrograms (mcg.) = 1/1,000,000 of a gram or International Units (I.U.), a standard measure of activity.

Claimed Benefits Of Taking Supplements: This section lists the reported good effects of taking a vitamin or mineral which go beyond general good health and the avoidance of deficiency symptoms. Many claims may be unproven or controversial. Some benefits may be reported only after people have taken doses which are much higher than the RDA's.

Reported Side Effects And Unsafe Dosages: This section discusses unwanted side effects and unsafe amounts of intake which have been reported for a vitamin or mineral. There is no guarantee that taking large amounts of a vitamin or mineral which are less than reported harmful levels will be completely safe or beneficial. New research can change the information reported about vitamins and minerals. Please, check carefully with your doctor for the most up-to-date information before you take any vitamin or mineral supplements in large amounts.

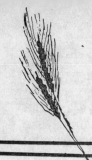

Vitamins

Vitamin A (Retinol, Carotene)

What It Does: Helps night vision . . . maintains smoothness, health and functions of the skin and areas of the body related to the skin, such as the mucous membranes of the mouth, throat, lungs, stomach, intestines and genital areas . . . helps build body protein and promotes growth of body tissues . . . stabilizes lysosomes, small structures within each body cell which defend against invaders.

Food Sources: Liver; especially cod liver oil, is the most concentrated source of vitamin A. Vitamin A is also found in eggs, whole milk products, broccoli, spinach, and other green, leafy vegetables. Carotene, which a healthy body can convert into vitamin A, is found in fruits and vegetables, especially yellow vegetables such as carrots. Many vitamins are partially destroyed by cooking, but carotene is released when vegetables are cooked. Thus, cooked vegetables are better sources of carotene than raw vegetables, as long as the juice is consumed.

How Long It Stays In Your Body: Vitamin A is a fat-soluble vitamin. It dissolves in body fat, and it can be stored for a long time, particularly in the liver. The liver can store several months' supply of vitamin A (about 200,000 IU). Water-soluble vitamins can be quickly flushed out of the body through the kidneys into the urine if you take too much. Fat-soluble vitamins like vitamin A may stay in the body for a long time at harmful levels if you take too much.

Deficiency Diseases And Symptoms: Night blindness or loss of vision in near darkness is the earliest symptom of a vitamin A deficiency. Other symptoms of vitamin A deficiency are dry, brittle hair, cracked, dry or blemished skin, itching or burning eyes, thickened eyelids, cloudy eye whites and eventually, in extreme cases, disintegration of the eyeball. In vitamin A deficiency, the lungs, digestive system and the urinary or reproductive systems may deteriorate. Victims may lose their sense of smell and experience softening of tooth enamel. Increased infections or difficulty in fighting infections may occur. Poor growth may be noticeable in children.

What Reduces, Destroys Or Increases It: Women taking birth control pills usually show an increase in levels of vitamin A in their blood of 30% to 80%. Smoking or drinking alcohol may destroy vitamin A or increase the body's need for vitamin A.

Long-term intestinal disease, which interferes with the absorption of vitamin A, can cause vitamin A deficiency even when vitamin A is present in the diet. Vitamins B2, B12, C and E aid in absorption of vitamin A.

Recommended Daily Dietary Allowance (RDA): Infants 1500 I.U.; children 2000 - 3500 I.U.; adult males 5000 I.U.; adult females 4000 I.U.; pregnant females 5000 I.U.; nursing mothers 6000 I.U.

Claimed Benefits Of Taking Supplements: Vitamin A may help in the treatment of acne, bronchial asthma, colds, conjunctivitis, emphysema, hyperthyroidism, glaucoma, measles, and migraines.

People with a slight deficiency of vitamin A may experience better night vision or smoother skin, with fewer blemishes and better overall health. Even in cases where people don't have gross deficiency symptoms, extra vitamin A supplementation is advised for people with diabetes and liver disease, because they may not have the ability to convert or utilize the vitamin efficiently.

A special water-soluble form of vitamin A should be given by intramuscular injection, by a physician, to people with long-term intestinal disease if the disease interferes with the absorption of fats and fat-soluble vitamins.

Vitamin A or beta-carotene may offer some degree of protection from cancer in statistical studies. The United States Government is now sponsoring a large study by the National Cancer Institute and Harvard University to get more information about the benefits of vitamin A in preventing cancer.

Unfortunately, a recent article in The New England Journal of Medicine reported that people who get cancer and those who don't get cancer had similar blood levels of carotene before cancer was detected.

Derivatives of vitamin A are used as acne treatments and experimental anticancer drugs.

Reported Side Effects And Unsafe Doses: Taking supplements of vitamin A close to the RDA is not reported to cause side effects in most people. Taking 20 times the RDA for one or two days may be used by physicians to restore levels in people who have symptoms of vitamin A deficiency. However, large doses of vitamin A are not advised for anyone else, and very large doses can be quite harmful and even poisonous. Eskimos and Arctic explorers avoid eating the poisonous livers of polar bears which contain millions of I.U.'s of vitamin A.

Adults taking repeated daily doses of around 10 times the RDA have reported harmful side effects. Similar harmful side effects have also been reported by adults taking over a million units of vitamin A in a single dose: buildup of pressure within the skull, vomiting, irritability, peeling of skin, loss of hair, dry skin and cracked lips. Infants that have been given large doses of vitamin A may suffer from itching, dehydration, muscle tremors, bulging fontanels or soft spots in the skull, and poor heart rhythm from high levels of blood calcium associated with vitamin A poisoning.

Women who use Accutane®, a drug derived from vitamin A, during pregnancy have a 20% chance of delivering a malformed child. Accutane®, and possibly vitamin A, can cause severe birth defects.

The symptoms of vitamin A deficiency are quite severe, and the possible harmful side effects from vitamin A overdoses are also quite severe. Most reports of vitamin A overdoses come from people who have taken 10 times the RDA or more for an extended period. Most people who don't have intestinal problems can avoid vitamin A deficiency and vitamin A overdose without risking serious side effects, by eating healthy amounts of fruits and vegetables, particularly yellow vegetables like carrots or squash which contain carotene. Anyone who takes a supplement of the active form of vitamin A should be cautious about taking more than the RDA.

The body makes vitamin A out of carotene. Excessive carotene which is found in plant sources may produce a different and less harmful side effect than large amounts of vitamin A. Large doses of carotene may cause the skin of some people to turn yellow or orange (for example, after drinking large amounts of carrot or tomato juice day after day).

Vitamin B12 (Cobalamin; Cyanocobalamin)

What It Does: Essential for: cell reproduction, growth and the manufacture of DNA and RNA which is the cells' genetic material . . . assists in the manufacture of the covering of the spinal cord and brain . . . helps convert folic acid and iron for the body's use . . . helps convert carbohydrates to fat . . . helps the body use fats, proteins and carbohydrates . . . may be important in maintaining fertility . . . promotes growth and appetite in children . . necessary for bone growth and repair.

Food Sources: Liver, meat, milk, dairy products, fish and eggs. Vitamin B12 is virtually absent in vegetables.

How Long It Stays In Your Body: Vitamin B12 is retained in the body longer than any other vitamin. Deficiency symptoms may not appear for months or even years after withdrawal of vitamin B12 from the diet.

Deficiency Diseases And Symptoms: Pernicious anemia is caused by vitamin B12 deficiency. The first symptoms are: depression, loss of appetite, fatigue and shortness of breath. Later, soreness of the mouth and tongue, diarrhea, weight gain, heart pain, pounding heartbeat and confusion may occur. Long-term deficiency may cause a deterioration of the nervous system with symptoms such as numbness and tingling of the feet, loss of reflexes, difficulty in walking, uncontrollable muscle movements, paralysis and psychosis. These latter symptoms involving the nervous system may be the only ones present if large amounts of folic acid are present in the diet, and B12 is deficient. For this reason, supplements of folic acid are limited by the U. S. Government to 800 mcg., a level which should allow for early detection of pernicious anemia in people who are deficient in vitamin B12.

People with pernicious anemia due to a lack of the "intrinsic factor", a substance made by the stomach that is necessary for B12 absorption through the intestines, need supplements by injection. For them, a dose of 100 micrograms is given 1 to 3 times weekly until levels are therapeutic (desired level). Then, a dose of 100 micrograms is given monthly. The need for these injections continues for life.

What Reduces, Destroys Or Increases It: Long-term intestinal diseases such as ileitis and the body's failure to make the "intrinsic factor" prevent the absorption of vitamin B12.

Aspirin and aspirin substitutes like acetaminophen, codeine, chloramphenicol, neomycin, oral contraceptives and calcium propionate (added to food to prevent spoilage) may reduce the amount of vitamin B12 available to the body. Excessively acidic or alkaline conditions in the intestines or a lack of calcium may interfere with the intestine's ability to absorb vitamin B12.

Recommended Daily Dietary Allowance (RDA): Infants .05 microgram_s (mcg.) - 1.5 mcg.; children 2.0 mcg. - 3.0 mcg.; adult males 3.0 mcg.; adult females 3.0 mcg.; pregnant women 4.0 mcg.; nursing mothers 4.0 mcg.

Claimed Benefits Of Taking Supplements: Absorption of B12 decreases with age. It is important that older people make sure that adequate B12 is available. B12 has been given for fatigue or a feeling of being "run-down".

Vegetarians, especially those who do not eat eggs or milk, may need supplements to prevent the development of pernicious anemia.

Children who appear to have "stunted" growth may benefit from additional B12. Studies have shown that B12 sometimes increases growth in children.

Reported Side Effects And Unsafe Doses: There is no evidence of vitamin B12 harm at doses usually taken. Preparations taken by mouth usually contain 25 to 250 micrograms, amounts which should be more than adequate.

Vitamin C (Ascorbic Acid; Sodium or Calcium Ascorbate; Antiscorbutic Acid)

What It Does: Essential for the formation and maintenance of intracellular ground substance and collagen, which form connective tissues in the body that hold the rest of the body together like threads and glue . . . strengthens immune mechanisms protecting the body from bacterial and viral infections . . . strengthens walls of blood vessels and reduces damage to them caused by aging or by artificial or natural chemical agents . . . reduces blood cholesterol and fat levels . . . promotes healthy gums by preventing tartar from forming . . . needed for proper function of glands regulating sex hormones . . . may increase fertility . . . can neutralize toxic or poisonous substances in the body . . . large amounts are used for protection by the body during periods of physical and emotional stress . . . helps in the body's absorption of iron . . . promotes wound healing . . . helps regulate normal body growth . . . necessary for proper function of adrenal glands.

Food Sources: Rose hips (berries found beneath the petals of a rosebud) and acerola cherries are the richest sources of Vitamin C. Green peppers, parsley, broccoli, brussels sprouts, cabbage and potatoes supply high levels of C. Fruits, especially citrus fruits, are good sources of vitamin C. Cooking causes 50% to 55% of vitamin C to be lost. If copper or iron utensils are used, the loss is greater. Fresh, refrigerated or frozen juices have higher amounts of vitamin C than canned juices.

How Long It Stays In Your Body: The body cannot make its own vitamin C in significant amounts. Small amounts are stored in the adrenal glands. It is thought that approximately 1500 mg. of ascorbic acid is maintained in the healthy person's body. For best functioning, the body's store should be kept full. Vitamin C is water soluble. If more is taken than the body can use or store, the extra amount is spilled into the urine within a few hours.

Studies show that only a small percentage of large doses of vitamin C above 1000 mg. at a time are absorbed into the body through the intestines.

Deficiency symptoms occur when less than 300 mg. are present in the body's stores or after 30 to 45 days without consuming vitamin C.

Deficiency Diseases And Symptoms: Vitamin C deficiency causes scurvy. Early signs of scurvy are bleeding under the skin, easy bruising, bleeding and swelling of the gums, tiredness and tooth and gum infections. Advance symptoms of scurvy include stomach and intestinal discomfort, body sores, fluid retention (edema), dry hair and skin, joint pain, depression and loss of teeth. Finally, death will occur as the connective tissues of the body deteriorate.

What Reduces, Destroys Or Increases It: Heat, oxygen and light destroy vitamin C in food. Fresh foods are best. Frozen foods are almost as good as fresh foods, but canned foods may have lost as much as 80% of the vitamin C they contained before processing. Lightly cooked foods contain more C than heavily cooked foods. Cooking in copper pots can destroy more vitamin C than cooking in other utensils.

Smoking one cigarette can destroy as much as 25 mg. of vitamin C. Aspirin causes vitamin C to be eliminated from the body. Oral contraceptives cause deficiencies of vitamin C, and very high levels of vitamin C can increase levels of estrogen, one of the components of some oral contraceptives. Illegal drugs, such as marijuana and cocaine, and some prescription drugs reduce vitamin C availability. Alcohol also inhibits absorption.

Bioflavonoids, found in the pulp and pith of citrus fruits, calcium and magnesium increase the actions of vitamin C. Small amounts of carbohydrates in the intestinal tract are needed for the absorption of vitamin C. Large doses of vitamin C may increase the activity of many acidic prescription drugs and decrease the activity of many alkaline prescription drugs such as amphetamines and tricyclic antidepressants.

Recommended Daily Dietary Allowance (RDA): Infants 35 mg.; children 45 mg.; adult males 50 - 60 mg.; adult females 50 - 60 mg.; pregnant women 70 - 80 mg.; nursing mothers 90 - 100 mg.

Claimed Benefits Of Taking Supplements: Vitamin C is claimed to cure, prevent or reduce the occurence of the common cold. Most studies show that taking large amounts of vitamin C may reduce the incidence of colds by 20% or 30% and that people who take large amounts of vitamin C have fewer cold symptoms than people who don't. Many medical doctors challenge the use of vitamin C in preventing or treating colds. They say that vitamin C either has little or no effect or that its effect is the same as that of an antihistamine in reducing cold symptoms but not in actually fighting the cold.

People who use vitamin C to fight colds usually report best results from increasing the amount of vitamin C taken immediately after the first symptoms of a cold appear. Many people like Dr. Linus Pauling, a Nobel prize-winning biochemist, advocate taking as much as

1000 mg. every hour and up to 20 grams per day to fight a cold or suppress its symptoms. When symptoms disappear under such a regimen, the infection may still be present; so vitamin C intake is gradually reduced over the next 10 days to prevent cold symptoms from returning.

One theory of how vitamin C helps fight colds and other viruses is that it increases the activity of the body's immune system. Studies show that vitamin C improves the ability of the body to produce interferon and to activate white blood cells which help defend the body from invaders.

Vitamin C may offer protection from poisonous substances. Nitrates and nitrites used in food preservation combine with amino acids in the body to form nitrosamines. Nitrosamines are thought to be cancer-causing substances. Vitamin C is thought to prevent this combination from taking place.

Ascorbic acid has been used in the treatment of mercury, lead and cadmium poisoning. Carbon monoxide, a poisonous gas given off by automobiles, cigarettes and malfunctioning heaters, attaches to red blood cells when it enters the body. Vitamin C pulls carbon monoxide from the red blood cells so that oxygen can be restored and carried to the body. Vitamin C may also play a role in reducing the toxic effects of certain drugs.

Some people have greater needs for vitamin C than others. Smokers and heavy alcohol drinkers need extra vitamin C. People with diabetes may need extra vitamin C. Diabetics may not be able to transport vitamin C into cells. This may contribute to the blood vessel damage that diabetics experience. People with arthritis who take large amounts of aspirin may be helped by taking extra vitamin C.

Recently a study at the University of Texas indicated that vitamin C may increase fertility in males by preventing the clumping of sperm, leaving more sperm available for fertilization. Extra vitamin C may be needed by women taking oral contraceptives.

Advancing age may be a good reason for C supplements. Vitamin C is an **antioxidant** that may slow down increased harmful peroxidation and free-radical formation in the elderly. It is thought that free-radicals play a major role in aging, heart disease, hardening of the arteries and cancer.

Vitamin C can play a role in the treatment or prevention of cancer. Terminal cancer patients, with cancer so advanced that other treatments had been abandoned, who were given vitamin C lived a few more months before dying than those not given vitamin C. <u>If you have cancer, do not stop or change the treatment prescribed by your physician, but you may want to discuss the benefits of vitamin C supplementation.</u> The National Academy of Science Committee On Diet, Nutrition And Cancer states: "Vitamin C can inhibit the formation of some carcinogens (cancer-causing substances) and that the consumption of vitamin C containing foods is associated with a lower risk of cancers of the stomach and esophagus."

Vitamin C deficiency is thought to be one factor in the development of heart disease. Reduction of cholesterol and the removal of plaque from artery walls are thought to be two possible beneficial effects of vitamin C. The antioxidant actions of vitamin C may also be helpful. These actions may be of greatest benefit when used with other nutrients such as vitamins A, E, B1, B5, B6, certain amino acids and the mineral selenium. <u>Again, you should see your physician before changing any treatment for heart disease or starting a multivitamin program.</u>

Fatigue may be related to low levels of vitamin C. The brain and spinal cord require vitamin C for proper function. People with the mental disorder schizophrenia have low levels of vitamin C in their blood, apparently because their bodies use up vitamin C at a higher than normal rate.

Vitamin C supplementation is reported to cut allergic and asthmatic attacks in half according to a controlled scientific study.

Vitamin C supplementation may help to lower eyeball pressure in glaucoma . . . reduce pain . . . reduce sensitivity to cold temperatures . . . have a natural laxative effect . . . fight tiredness . . . help broken bones heal quickly . . . and fight stress.

Vitamin C is necessary for fast healing of sunburn, wounds and surgical incisions. Taking extra vitamin C before and after these injuries is proven to help the healing process.

Reported Side Effects And Unsafe Doses: Vitamin C is claimed to be one of the least toxic vitamins. Studies indicate that large doses of more than 500 mg per day of vitamin C, which in small doses is an antioxidant, can, paradoxically, cause opposite results, harmful free radical formation and peroxidation.

Taking large doses of vitamin C to suppress a cold can cause serious complications. Viral meningitis or Reye's syndrome with symptoms like extreme headache, fever, vomiting or coma may occur because vitamin C may fool the body's defenses and let a suppressed virus linger long enough in the body to get into the nervous system. The same cautions that apply to taking large doses of aspirin in cases of viral attacks should also apply to vitamin C.

Some vitamin C formulations contain sodium (sodium ascorbate) or calcium (calcium ascorbate). People on low-sodium diets should avoid taking sodium ascorbate. People receiving digitalis or other heart medication should not take calcium ascorbate, since irregular heartbeats may occur.

Vitamin C in the form of ascorbic acid can burn the stomach and cause nausea, indigestion, diarrhea or stomach ulcers. Vitamin C in the form of ascorbic acid should always be taken with food or with a large amount of water and an antacid.

Diabetics taking oral drugs to lower their blood sugar and heart patients taking anticoagulants should not take vitamin C without the supervision of a physician, because it may block the action of these drugs. Vitamin C taken with sulfa-drugs may cause the formation of harmful crystals in the kidneys. Vitamin C may block some of the activity of fertility drugs and the drug disulfiram (Antabuse) which is given to alcoholics. High doses of vitamin C may cause false readings in laboratory tests for blood sugar levels. High doses of vitamin C can cause false negative results when testing for hidden blood in stool specimens.

High doses of vitamin C may increase the body's need for folic acid and vitamin B12. Vitamin C increases the absorption of iron into the body. Large doses of vitamin C interfere with the formation of hemoglobin for red blood cells by reducing the absorption and use of copper which is important in the formation of hemoglobin. People taking large doses of Vitamin C should eat foods which are high in copper and have regular blood tests to see if they have become anemic. People who take large doses of vitamin C may build up a tolerance to it which works against many of the claimed benefits of taking high doses.

Symptoms of vitamin C deficiency may appear when there is a rapid decrease in large doses of vitamin C which have been taken. This "rebound effect" may cause aches and pains and increase the number of colds. People who have been taking large doses of vitamin C temporarily should cut down gradually to avoid the "rebound effect". "Rebound" vitamin C deficiency can occur in infants born to women who have taken high doses of vitamin C.

High doses of vitamin C may cause high levels of uric acid in the blood. Some studies indicate that large doses of vitamin C can create conditions which might increase the rate of oxalate kidney or urinary tract stone formation, but other studies indicate that people who take large doses of vitamin C do not have an increase in the rate of stone formation. Large doses of vitamin C may cause the destruction of red blood cells in victims of the G-6-PD enzyme deficiency disease. Taking high doses of vitamin C may increase the chance of developing aortic aneurysm (ballooning and possible rupture of the largest blood vessel in the body).

Vitamin D (Calciferol; Viosterol; Ergosterol; Sunshine Vitamin)

What It Does: Essential for the absorption and regulation of calcium and phosphorus which are necessary for strong bones and teeth . . . helps the body use magnesium . . . helps in forming vitamin A . . . needed for muscle tone . . .helps kidney function.

Food Sources: The best source is the sun's action on the skin which forms vitamin D. Fish and fish liver oils are rich sources of this vitamin. Other food sources are liver, eggs and milk which has been fortified with vitamin D.

How Long It Stays In Your Body: Vitamin D is fat soluble. It can be absorbed through the intestines along with dietary fat. Inactive forms of vitamin D are stored in the liver and converted into active forms as needed. The liver can store several month's supply of vitamin D.

Deficiency Diseases And Symptoms: Vitamin D deficiency causes poor bone growth or poor formation of bones. This condition is known as rickets in children or osteomalacia in adults. Osteomalacia or rickets may occur when: (1) exposure of the skin to sunlight is low (2) vitamin D in the diet is low (3) the body is not able to change the inactive form of vitamin D, which is stored in the body, to the active form which the body can use (4) there is a problem with the absorption of vitamin D into the body.

Symptoms of vitamin D deficiency in children are not easily recognized at first. Infants may be restless and sleep poorly. The bones surrounding the soft spots on the head may take longer than usual to come together. The infant may take longer to learn to sit or crawl.

As a child with vitamin D deficiency becomes older, there may be pain when walking, and obvious deformities of the bone, such as knock knees or bowlegs, are likely to develop. In adults, early symptoms of vitamin D deficiency may be constipation, muscle weakness, cramps and nervousness. Bone cracks may be seen on x-rays as bones lose minerals which are needed to maintain strength. Vitamin D deficiency may contribute to osteoporosis and other diseases involving loss of minerals from bone. Vitamin D deficiency may cause hypocalcemia (low levels of calcium, since vitamin D is necessary for the absorption of calcium into the body). Low levels of calcium in the blood may cause cramps or muscle spasms.

What Reduces, Destroys, Or Increases It: Anything that blocks sunshine from penetrating the skin will reduce the amount of vitamin D that the body makes. Vitamin D is made by the action of the sun's ultraviolet rays on the skin. The ultraviolet rays only penetrate the atmosphere when the sun is high on the horizon. Very little ultraviolet light reaches the earth's surface in northern latitudes in the winter months even when the sun is at its highest point at mid-day. On the other hand, when the sun is high on the horizon in the summer, full exposure of the skin to sun in sunbathing produces a very large amount of vitamin D in just a few minutes. People who have been overexposed to direct sunlight to the point of receiving sunburns often suffer symptoms of vitamin D overdose, like chills and lightheadedness.

Vitamin D is stored in the body in an inactive form. Smoking interferes with the activation of vitamin D which has been stored in the body. Anticonvulsant drugs may cause the breakdown of vitamin D. Barbiturate drugs reduce the effectiveness of vitamin D. Mineral oil based laxatives and the drug cholestyramine interfere with the absorption of vitamin D through the intestines. Liver, gall bladder and intestinal diseases may interfere with the absorption of vitamin D or prevent the body from using vitamin D properly. Thiamine, niacin and vitamin A help the body tolerate overdoses of vitamin D. Vitamin C helps prevent the breakdown of vitamin D in the body.

Recommended Daily Dietary Allowance (RDA): Infants 400 I.U.; children 400 I.U.; adult males 200 - 400 I.U.; adult females 200 - 400 I.U.; pregnant women 400 - 600 I.U.; nursing mothers 400 - 600 I.U.

Claimed Benefits Of Taking Supplements: The requirement for vitamin D decreases when people reach their full growth. However, as people grow older, it is important to receive the RDA of this vitamin to prevent osteoporosis or bone loss. Osteoporosis is a serious problem in the elderly, especially in aging women after the menopause when calcium loss from the bones increases dramatically.

Vitamin D supplements may help counteract some of the side effects of therapy with steroid hormones like cortisone. Vitamin D is sometimes used by physicians to counteract overstimulation of the parathyroid glands which often occurs when steroid drugs are taken.

Vitamin D supplementation may help to control epileptic seizures, but this treatment is unproven.

Reported Side Effects And Unsafe Doses: Vitamin D is one of the few vitamins which is reported to be harmful when doses only slightly above the RDA are taken. If you've ever been sunburned, you have probably suffered from vitamin D overdose. Symptoms are: unusual thirst, itching, stomach or intestinal discomfort, chills, lightheadedness, headache, loss of balance, ringing in the ears, vomiting, diarrhea, constipation, pain in the muscles and bones, decreased sex drive, high blood pressure, runny nose, inflammation of the pancreas and, rarely, severe mental illness. Vitamin D overdose can cause death from kidney or heart failure. Long-term overdoses of vitamin D, which might occur from taking too much in the form of supplements, may include sore eyes, sensitivity to light, increased urination, painful urination, bone loss, calcium deposits in the liver, lungs, kidneys, stomach or blood vessels.

Fair-skinned people should be careful about sunbathing for more than 15 minutes when the sun is high on the horizon during the summer months if they don't have a tan. Fair-skinned people who do have tans should be careful about sunbathing in strong direct sunlight for more than one hour. Dark-skinned people can also suffer from sunburn after longer exposure than fair-skinned people. Whenever sunburn occurs, symptoms of vitamin D overdose may be present.

The use of vitamin D and magnesium containing antacids may lead to high levels of magnesium in the body. Vitamin D may cause heart irregularities in people who are taking digitalis or verapamil. People with low parathyroid gland function who take thiazide diuretics may suffer from high blood levels of calcium when vitamin D supplements are taken. Overdoses of vitamin D taken in pregnancy may cause birth defects like aortic stenosis or hypoparathyroidism.

Vitamin E (d-alpha-tocopherol; other tocopherols)

What It Does: Vitamin E is an antioxidant. It protects the body from damage by oxidation and free-radicals. Vitamin E stabilizes cell membranes . . . helps in the formation of red blood cells, muscles and other tissues. It protects red blood cells against rupturing. Vitamin E helps the body use vitamin A . . . protects against unwanted blood clots . . . protects against damage which can be caused by polyunsaturated fats . . . plays a role in the function of the body's immune system by helping to produce antibodies and helping to activate white blood cells.

Food Sources: Whole-grain products are rich in vitamin E. Vegetable oils and margarine contain high levels of vitamin E before processing but may contain low levels of vitamin E after processing. Cottonseed oil contains more vitamin E after processing than other vegetable oils. The outer leaves of green vegetables are good sources of vitamin E. Milk, almonds, peanuts, pecans, soybeans, eggs and meat also contain vitamin E.

How Long It Stays In Your Body: Vitamin E is a fat-soluble vitamin, and it can build up in the body indefinitely if large doses are taken. However, vitamin E which is stored in the body is not retained by the body over a long period of time. Half of the body's stored vitamin E may be used up in two or three weeks.

Deficiency Diseases And Symptoms: Vitamin E is present in a variety of foods, so obvious deficiency symptoms usually are seen only in infants and in people with intestinal diseases that cause poor absorption of fats. When vitamin E is deficient, red blood cells in adults become fragile. Muscles, including the muscles of the small intestine, may deteriorate. Permanent damage to reproduction organs and sterility can occur. In newborn infants, especially in premature babies of low birth weight, vitamin E deficiency may cause hemolytic anemia.

What Reduces, Destroys Or Increases It: The need for vitamin E increases when the intake of polyunsaturated fatty acids increases. Polyunsaturated fatty acids are found in margarine, shortening and vegetable oils which also contain vitamin E, but vitamin E can be destroyed by heat that is used in processing these foods.

Chlorine, found in chlorinated drinking water, reduces the availability of vitamin E in the body as vitamin E neutralizes the chlorine. Vitamin E is destroyed by "ferric" iron compounds like those found in some iron supplements. Copper also destroys vitamin E. Oral contraceptives reduce the amount of vitamin E available in the body. Illnesses which cause poor intestinal absorption reduce the absorption of vitamin E. Canning food destroys over 75% of the vitamin E content of vegetables.

Many vitamins and minerals are more beneficial to the body when given with vitamin E. Vitamins A, the B-complex, C, manganese, phosphorus, selenium and inositol are found to have greater effect in the body in combination with E.

Recommended Daily Dietary Allowance (RDA): Infants 4 - 6 I.U.; children 7 - 10 I.U.; adult males 12 - 15 I.U.; adult females 12 I.U.; pregnant women 15 I.U.; nursing mothers 16 I.U.

Claimed Benefits Of Taking Supplements: Vitamin E is thought to reduce the damage from oxygen therapy in low birth weight infants. Vitamin E is also thought to decrease a tendency toward hemolytic anemia in infants, especially low birth weight infants. Three to five I.U. given by mouth is recommended for low birth weight infants. Vitamin E is used to prevent or treat the eye disease, retinopathy of prematurity. Higher doses are no more helpful in treating this disease than the recommended doses and can be harmful.

Much vitamin E is destroyed in polyunsaturated fats which have undergone chemical processing under extreme heat to prevent them from hardening. The body's need for vitamin E is largely dependent upon the amount of polyunsaturated fats in the diet. People who consume large quantities of chemically processed vegetable oils, which are high in polyunsaturated fats, may need additional supplements of vitamin E.

Vitamin E has an anticoagulant effect. It has been used to prevent blood clots and pulmonary embolism in bedridden patients and to treat people with poor circulation in the legs (intermittent claudication) who have a tendency to have leg cramps and form blood clots in the legs.

Vitamin E has been used to ease the "hot flashes" and other uncomfortable side effects associated with menopause. Vitamin E has been used to reduce the non-cancerous swellings found in fibrocystic breast disease. It has also been shown to fight pollutants, boost the immune system, relieve muscle cramping, and maintain the health of the eyes, lungs, heart, and skeletal muscles.

Less well documented claims for vitamin E include: reduced rates of aging, reduction in symptoms associated with hardening of the arteries or heart disease, and fewer skin wrinkles.

Reported Side Effects And Unsafe Doses: Most of the medical research on vitamin E indicates that it is a relatively safe vitamin to take in moderate doses. Unfortunately, there is one study which is so alarming in its findings that it indicates that vitamin E taken in large doses may be very harmful. This study by Enstrom and Pauling showed, with statistical significance, that people who took high doses of vitamin E over a long period of time had higher death rates than those who took moderate doses of vitamin E. People in this study who took 1000 I.U. or more daily, or others who did not take any vitamin E supplements, had twice the death rate of those who took lower doses of vitamin E or others who did not take any vitamin E supplements. **People should exercise great caution in taking large doses of vitamin E until this study can be confirmed or disproven by additional research.**

Vitamin E is routinely given to low-birth weight newborn infants; but recently, 43 low-birth weight newborn infants died, apparently as a result of receiving E-Ferol, a form of vitamin E, intravenously. The dangers of intravenous administration of vitamin E are now under study by the Food and Drug Administration.

Infants given high doses of vitamin E often develop bacterial or fungal infections or necrotising enterocolitis, an intestinal disease.

Taking vitamin E in doses larger than the RDA is reported to sometimes cause indigestion, headache, enlarged breasts in men and women, reduced sexual function, fatigue, high blood pressure, jaundice or yellow skin, intestinal distress, blood clots in the lungs and legs and destruction of intestinal tissue. Vitamin E seems to slow down metabolism and cause longer running times in long-distance runners. Large amounts of vitamin E may cause tiredness, high blood pressure, muscle weakness, and interference with vitamin K, thyroid, adrenal and pituitary hormone function. Vitamin E may increase the effects of oral anticoagulants.

Vitamin K

What It Does: Helps the blood to clot . . . helps stop bleeding . . . essential for the production of prothrombin and other blood clotting factors . . . converts glucose into glycogen for storage in the liver.

Food Sources: Green, leafy vegetables, fruits, cereals, dairy products and meats are all rich sources of vitamin K. Vitamin K is also supplied by micro-organisms living in the intestines.

How Long It Stays In Your Body: Vitamin K is a fat-soluble vitamin. Most of the body's stores of vitamin K are found in the liver. Small amounts can be found in the kidneys and in the bone marrow. Deficiency symptoms can appear within four weeks after the onset of intestinal problems which interfere with the absorption of vitamin K.

What Reduces, Destroys Or Increases It: Mineral oil based laxatives interfere with the absorption of vitamin K. Aspirin and anticoagulants of the warfarin class (Coumadin®, Dicumarol®) interfere with the action of vitamin K. Oral contraceptives can cause a build-up of vitamin K in the body.

Deficiency Diseases And Symptoms: Deficiency symptoms include excessive bleeding, easy bruising and, finally, uncontrollable bleeding. Deficiency symptoms usually will not occur when there is a dietary deficiency, because of the production of vitamin K in the intestines by micro-organisms. Vitamin K deficiency symptoms usually happen when intestinal disease interferes with the absorption of vitamin K into the body.

Recommended Daily Dietary Allowance (RDA):
Infants 10 - 20 micrograms, mcg.; children 15 -100 mcg.; adults 70 - 140 mcg.

Claimed Benefits Of Taking Supplements: Newborn infants lack vitamin K. In fact, they are routinely given vitamin K shots. They can benefit from vitamin K supplements until milk or milk-based formula has been consumed for one week and friendly intestinal microbes have become established. Pregnant mothers may benefit from taking vitamin K to protect them from excessive bleeding following delivery. People on diets containing few vegetables or people with intestinal problems also may find taking this vitamin helpful.

Reported Side Effects And Unsafe Doses: One form of vitamin K, menadione, from animal sources may cause liver damage if taken in high doses. Another form of vitamin K, phylloquinone, from plant sources is less apt to cause liver damage. Large amounts of vitamin K taken during pregnancy can cause jaundice in newborn infants.

Biotin

What It Does: Helps the body use protein, polyunsaturated fatty acids and other fats . . . helps maintain the function of skin, hair, oil and sweat glands, nerves, bone marrow, ovaries, testes and liver.

Food Sources: Biotin is widely distributed in many plant and animal foods. Most of the biotin in wheat and raw egg whites is in a "bound" or not usable form. Good sources of biotin are rye, brewer's yeast, liver, eggs, mung bean sprouts, dairy products, brown rice, nuts, chicken, corn, soybeans, fish (especially tuna, clams and mackerel), dried peas, butter and cauliflower.

How Long It Stays In Your Body: Biotin is water soluble, but it isn't eliminated from the body as quickly as many other water-soluble vitamins. Some biotin is stored in the liver. Some biotin is manufactured by micro-organisms living in the intestines.

Deficiency Diseases And Symptoms: Dry, red, scaly changes in the skin and hair loss are among early deficiency signs. There may also be a lack of appetite, nausea, vomiting, lack of energy, sleeplessness, depression and muscle pains. If the deficiency goes without treatment, severe heart pains and paralysis may occur.

In infants, usually those less than six months old, skin diseases have been associated with biotin deficiency.

Biotin deficiencies are rare. "Egg-white injury" may occur if the diet includes a large number of raw eggs which are deficient in usable biotin. Deficiency symptoms have also been associated with the use of antibiotics which may kill micro-organisms that manufacture biotin in the intestinal tract.

What Reduces, Destroys Or Increases It: Antibiotics, including sulfa drugs, or intestinal disease, can kill micro-organisms in the intestine which manufacture biotin. Alcohol destroys biotin in the body. Eating rancid fats or excessive amounts of choline reduces the stores of biotin in the liver. Saccharin can block the action of biotin. Riboflavin, niacin, pantothenic acid, vitamin B6, vitamin B12, vitamin A, vitamin D, growth hormone and testosterone are reported to increase the actions of biotin.

Recommended Daily Dietary Allowance (RDA): There is no official RDA for biotin, but the Food and Nutrition Board has suggested the following daily levels as being safe and adequate for human nutrition: adults 100 - 200 micrograms, mcg.; children under 12, 35 -120 mcg.; children over 12, 100 - 200 mcg.

Claimed Benefits Of Taking Supplements: Biotin is a useful addition to infant formulas, because biotin-manufacturing bacteria may not become established in the intestinal tract of infants until several days after birth.

There are indications that biotin lotions or ointments applied to the scalp may delay the development of pattern-baldness.

Reported Side Effects And Unsafe Doses: Unknown.

Choline

What It Does: Forms part of nervous system transmitter acetylcholine . . . necessary for proper liver and gallbladder function . . . important for immune system development . . . makes fatty acids usable by cells . . . helps in transportation of substances across cell walls . . needed for healthy kidneys . . . with inositol, manufactures lecithin in the body . . . needed for manufacture of thyroid hormones.

Food Sources: Lecithin, soybeans, eggs, fish, liver and wheat germ are rich sources of choline. Green vegetables, peanuts, brewer's yeast and sunflower seeds are other good sources of choline.

How Long It Stays In Your Body: Choline is absorbed through the intestinal wall; so intestinal diseases which interfere with absorption can reduce the amount of choline available. The body can make choline; however, the exact amount is not known. In emergency situations, an amino acid (serine) is capable of producing choline if the diet contains enough protein. More research is needed to discover storage and elimination patterns of choline.

Deficiency Diseases And Symptoms: Choline is widely distributed in many plant and animal foods. Severe deficiencies in humans are rare. Most of the research concerning choline deficiencies has been with laboratory animals. Choline withdrawal from the diet causes fat to build up in the liver within one or two days. Fatty cysts form in the liver. The liver loses its ability to convert harmful substances to harmless substances, and poisons build up in the body.

Rats fed a choline-deficient diet were found to develop

cancerous tumors. Another group given choline supplements did not develop the tumors. Animal offspring born of choline-deficient mothers have poor resistance to diseases because of poorly developed immune systems.

Other signs of choline deficiency are high blood pressure, bleeding stomach ulcers, noises in the ears, dizziness, sleeplessness, and vision difficulties.

What Reduces, Destroys Or Increases It: Diets low in dietary fiber and high in sugar promote the growth of micro-organisms in the intestines that consume choline, and reduce the growth of micro-organisms that produce choline or help choline to be absorbed through the intestinal wall into the body. The consumption of alcohol depletes choline supplies and causes fatty degeneration of the liver. Pantothenic acid, vitamin B12, folic acid, inositol and methionine, an amino acid, are necessary for choline to work properly in the body.

Recommended Daily Dietary Allowance (RDA): The RDA for choline has not been established by the Food and Nutrition Board. It is thought that a normal diet will contain between 400 and 1000 mg. per day.

Claimed Benefits Of Taking Supplements: Choline and inositol manufacture lecithin in the body. Lecithin is thought to have cholesterol- reducing properties. Although not proven, Alzheimer's disease, a disease affecting the memory in elderly people, may be slowed by supplementing the diet with lecithin. Choline by itself is thought to improve memory in normal people.

Choline supplements are reported to help control blood pressure. In one study, one-third of a group of patients with high blood pressure had their blood pressure return to normal after receiving choline supplements. When the supplements were discontinued, their blood pressure rose once again. Additional studies are needed to confirm that choline was responsible. <u>Anyone with high blood pressure should consult with his physician before changing prescribed treatment.</u>

Approximately 10% of people with mental illness who receive antipsychotic drugs such as Thorazine® or other phenothiazines for a long period develop a degenerative condition called tardive dyskinesia. Victims of tardive dyskinesia suffer from uncontrollable muscle movements. Physicians who treat mental illness with both antipsychotic drugs and large doses of vitamins, including choline, report that symptoms of tardive dyskinesia are absent among their patients.

Choline may play a role in fertility. A study shows that choline supplements in feed can increase the sizes of litters in some farm animals.

Glaucoma and kidney damage have also been treated with choline.

Reported Side Effects And Unsafe Doses: Choline supplements taken in doses greater than 50 mg. may cause diarrhea if the supplement was taken in the form of choline bitartrate. Choline chloride or choline hydrochloride is not reported to cause diarrhea when taken in large doses. Choline supplements may cause a fishy smell in the stool. Yogurt or extra dietary fiber may decrease the odor if it occurs.

Large doses of choline may cause deficiencies of vitamin B6. Large doses of choline may contribute to osteoporosis, bone degeneration common in older people, especially women. Choline seems to increase the uptake of phosphorus into the bones, and large doses may cause excessive uptake of phosphorus which may drive calcium out of the bones. If large doses of choline are taken, more calcium may be needed to maintain a proper calcium-phosphorus balance. <u>Caution! Choline should not be given to people who have manic-depressive psychosis, since substances which may increase acetylcholine formation tend to worsen this mental illness.</u>

Folic Acid

What It Does: Essential for red blood cell production . . . controls the development of nerve cells in the unborn child. . . helps produce DNA and RNA (genetic material) . . . helps bacteria in the intestines manufacture choline . . . helps activate enzymes responsible for the division of body cells. . . necessary for the maintenance of the nervous system, intestinal tract, white blood cells and sex organs. . . essential for red blood cell production. . . increases appetite . . . helps protein metabolism . . . needed by the body for proper use of sugar and amino acids . . . may help prevent graying of the hair.

Food Sources: Yeast, liver, lima beans, whole-grain products, leafy green vegetables, asparagus, beans, turnips, peanuts, oats, potatoes, oranges.

How Long It Stays In Your Body: Folic acid is a water-soluble vitamin. It may be stored in small amounts in the liver. Extra amounts of folic acid beyond the body's needs are usually excreted through the kidneys into the urine within 24 hours. Deficiency symptoms may occur after 100 days of low folic acid intake.

Deficiency Diseases And Symptoms: Folic acid deficiency causes an anemia similar to pernicious anemia. Early symptoms may be depression, loss of appetite, dizziness, fatigue and shortness of breath. Severe or prolonged deficiency may cause soreness of the mouth and tongue, diarrhea, heart pain, pounding heartbeat and confusion. The nervous system symptoms which are found in pernicious anemia are absent in the anemia caused by folic acid deficiency. Folic acid deficiency may sometimes be caused by intestinal disease which interferes with the body's ability to absorb folic acid. Folic acid should be supplemented by injection in cases of intestinal disease which interferes with absorption. Folic acid deficiency during pregnancy can cause hemorrhaging after delivery, premature delivery, and possible brain damage in the fetus and possible birth defects like spina bifida.

What Reduces, Destroys Or Increases It: Folic acid dissolves in cooking water when foods are heated. Cooking in copper pots or leaving food in copper pots after cooking destroys folic acid in the cooking water. Alcohol reduces the absorption of folic acid through the intestines. Oral contraceptives, aspirin, or aspirin substitutes such as acetaminophen (Tylenol®), Dilantin®, primidone, phenobarbital, methotrexate, pyrimethamine, and triamterene reduce the amount of folic acid available in the body. Both vitamin C deficiency and high doses of vitamin C have been reported to increase the body's need for folic acid.

Recommended Daily Dietary Allowance (RDA): Infants 30-45 micrograms mcg.; children 100-300 mcg.; adult males 400 mcg.; adult females 400 mcg.; pregnant females 800 mcg.; nursing mothers 500 mcg.

Claimed Benefits Of Taking Supplements: Folic acid deficiency is strongly suspected as a cause of birth defects. Adequate supplementation of folic acid is highly recommended for pregnant women or women who wish to become pregnant.

The FDA Consumer is an authoritative government publication. Recently, the FDA Consumer interviewed a Dr. Roe who has studied the effects of oral contraceptives on nutrients. Dr. Roe feels that folic acid is generally deficient in the American diet unless people eat substantial amounts of organ meat, dark-green leafy vegetables, or fortified breakfast cereals. Dr. Roe states that dysplasia of the cervix (abnormal development of the neck of the womb), which sometimes occurs with oral contraceptive use, improves when the victims take folic acid supplements. The article goes on to state: "Because pregnant women are predisposed to folate (folic acid) deficiency the labeling of OC's (oral contraceptives) advises that if a woman becomes pregnant shortly after stopping the pill she may have a greater chance of developing a folate deficiency and its complications." Folic acid helps hormones like estradiol and testosterone work effectively.

Older people, especially those over 70 years of age, are thought to have lower-than-normal folic acid levels, perhaps because of absorption problems. In one study, a group of elderly patients who had no obvious malnutrition experienced improvements in vision with folic acid supplementation.

Studies by Kurt A. Oster, M. D., and others indicate that large doses of folic acid (as much as 80 mg. per day) may be helpful in the treatment and prevention of diabetes and heart disease. Larger, controlled studies are necessary to confirm these small studies and reports of clinical experience.

High uric acid levels in diabetics are reported to be lowered by high doses of folic acid. Uric acid levels are reported to rise once again when folic acid supplementation is stopped.

One cardiologist who treats his heart patients with large doses of folic acid reports that no one in his study group who maintained certain blood levels of folic acid suffered heart attacks. He reports that in 80 out of 100 patients treated with high doses of folic acid the progress of coronary heart disease has been stopped, and in some cases the reported symptoms of coronary heart disease have diminished among his patients. Another medical doctor connected with this study states that folic acid may stop the progress of coronary heart disease by neutralizing xanthine oxidase and by restoring plasmalogin which repairs damage to arteries and helps stop the fatty buildup which is found in hardening of the arteries.

Treating diabetes and coronary heart disease with high doses of folic acid is a new and experimental therapy. Please consult your physician before changing any established treatment program for diabetes or coronary heart disease.

Reported Side Effects And Unsafe Doses: Doses of 1000 mcg. or more of folic acid per day may hide the symptoms of pernicious anemia which is caused by vitamin B12 deficiency. Therefore, the government has decreed that a prescription be required for doses over 800 mcg. per tablet. Skin rashes are the only reported side effect of moderately high folic acid intake among healthy people. Doses of folic acid of more than 10 times the RDA may cause nerve damage. Folic acid can block the action of sulfa drugs which are used to treat urinary tract infections and certain other conditions. People with a medical history of convulsive disorders such as epilepsy or certain types of hormone-related cancer should not take high doses of folic acid which may worsen these conditions. Please consult your physician before taking folic acid supplements if you have these conditions.

Inositol

What It Does: Combines with choline to form lecithin to break down fat and cholesterol . . . necessary for healthy hair and skin . . . necessary for vitamin B5 function . . . improves muscle tone and function . . . aids nervous system function.

Food Sources: Organ meats, yeast, beans, whole-grain products, peanuts and citrus fruits.

How Long It Stays In Your Body: Micro-organisms in the intestines of a healthy body produce large amounts of inositol. This makes it difficult for scientists to determine how long inositol is stored in the body.

Deficiency Diseases And Symptoms: Eczema, a condition causing dry, scaly patches on the skin, has been linked to inositol deficiency. Loss of hair has also been connected with inositol deficiency in animal studies. Other deficiency symptoms include eye abnormalities, high blood cholesterol and constipation.

What Reduces, Destroys Or Increases It: Mineral oil, antibiotics or intestinal disease may reduce the body's production or absorption of inositol in the intestines. Caffeine interferes with the body's use of inositol. Biotin, choline and vitamin E are needed for inositol to be used most effectively in the body.

Recommended Daily Dietary Allowance (RDA): There is no RDA for inositol, because inositol is not officially considered to be a vitamin. Nevertheless, inositol is generally recognized to have many vitamin-like qualities and to be important in human nutrition.

Claimed Benefits Of Taking Supplements: May help reduce levels of blood cholesterol . . . may help to break down fatty deposits in the liver which are present in liver diseases like cirrhosis . . . may have a slight inhibitory effect on bladder cancer . . . may be helpful in retarding the development of baldness . . .may increase the anxiety reducing properties of niacin . . . protects kidneys, liver, and heart. Inositol and vitamin E may help reduce damage to the nervous system caused by muscular dystrophy.

Reported Side Effects And Unsafe Doses: No short-term side effects have been reported in experimental studies using up to 3 grams per person per day.

Niacin (Vitamin B3; Nicotinic Acid; Niacinamide; Nicotinamide)

What It Does: Helps break down food to provide energy for the body . . . involved in energy transfer systems within the body . . . helps activate many enzymes . . . improves circulation . . . helps metabolize proteins, carbohydrates and fats . . . helps the body make certain hormones.

Food Sources: Yeast, fish, poultry, liver, meat, whole-grain products (except corn which contains an inactive form of niacin), peanuts, potatoes, beans, mushrooms.

How Long It Stays In Your Body: Niacin is water soluble, and the body cannot store it for long periods. When large amounts of niacin beyond the body's needs are taken, most is flushed out through the kidneys in the urine in a few hours.

Deficiency Diseases And Symptoms: Pellagra is the disease caused by niacine deficiency. Symptoms of pellagra appear in three body systems: the skin, the nervous system and the digestive system.

Early in the nineteenth century many cases of pellagra occurred in the United States, particularly in the South. Medical students during this period learned that the classic symptoms of pellagra were the three D's, "dementia, dermatitis and diarrhea."

Pellagra is associated with diets which are high in corn, white rice or unenriched, refined white flour. In the 1930's and 1940's pellagra became a rare disease in the United States as bakeries were required by law to add niacin to white bread, thus "enriching" it.

The earliest symptoms of pellagra are nervousness, insomnia, depression, bad breath, irritability, headaches or fatigue. Later, skin, mouth and other mucous membrane sores appear. There may be a skin rash resembling heat rash with painful red spots. Skin may have a red appearance like sunburn. Other early signs include nausea, loss of appetite, and muscular weakness.

In the later stages of the disease after prolonged or severe niacin deficiency, people may have hallucinations or other signs of severe schizophrenia-like mental illness. The skin may become dry, scaly and inflexible. The tongue may become red, sore and swollen. Sores may develop a grayish color and have a bad odor. Diarrhea, which is particularly dangerous in infants, develops. Finally, the lining of the stomach develops ulcers and bleeds. Without treatment at this point, death soon occurs.

What Reduces, Destroys Or Increases It: Cooking and soaking food in water cause niacin to be lost. Milling grain to produce white rice or white flour eliminates most of the niacin found in the grain. Sulfa drugs and other antibiotics, sleeping pills, alcohol and coffee reduce niacin in the body. Physical exercise and emotional stress increase requirements for carbohydrates and for niacin which is necessary for the body to use them.

Thiamine, riboflavin, and pyridoxine help the body convert tryptophan, an amino acid found in protein, into niacin. Many other vitamins work with niacin in the body and help the body use it efficiently.

Oral contraceptives increase the effects of niacin in the body.

Recommended Daily Dietary Allowance (RDA):
Infants 6 mg. - 8 mg.; children 9 mg. - 16 mg.; adult males 16 mg. - 18 mg.; adult females 13 mg. - 15 mg.; pregnant women 15 mg. - 17 mg.; nursing mothers 18 mg. - 20 mg.

Claimed Benefits Of Taking Supplements: Large doses (500-1000 mg three times per day) of niacin are useful in the treatment of schizophrenia. A small minority of psychiatrists use it as a treatment of first choice, but most psychiatrists think it isn't a reliable treatment. Accurate, controlled studies by Hoffer and Osmond with the provincial mental hospital patients of Saskatchewan in the 1950's prove the effectiveness of this treatment, but additional, controlled studies are needed to compare its overall effectiveness to other treatments. In many schizophrenics, it appears to be better than treatment with powerful tranquilizers, and it has fewer severe side effects. Many schizoid personalities or moderately severe long-term, chronic paranoid schizophrenics, for which it works best, improve dramatically after taking 1500-3000 mg. of niacin in 3 daily doses of 500-1000 mg/dose according to controlled studies. Niacin may help schizophrenics by increasing the body's production of serotonin, a nervous system hormone or by helping to rid the body of byproducts of faulty neurohormone metabolism.

Niacin, other B vitamins and vitamin C may be useful in preventing the development of tardive dyskinesia in mental patients who are taking powerful phenothiazine tranquilizers such as Thorazine®. Tardive dyskinesia is an irreversible deterioration of the central nervous system which causes uncontrollable muscle spasms in approximately 10% of the people who take phenothiazine tranquilizers over a long period of time. There have been no controlled studies in this area, but physicians who use both large doses of vitamins, including niacin, and powerful tranquilizers in their psychiatric practices for treatment of mental illness have reported seeing no cases of tardive dyskinesia among patients who have taken large doses of both niacin and other vitamins and phenothiazine tranquilizers for many years.

Niacin has been used to help the recovery of drug users who have taken LSD or other drugs which may cause hallucinations. Although there are no controlled studies in this area, some physicians have reported that drug abusers who have taken a "bad trip" often return to normal within one hour of taking one or more grams of niacin.

Niacin has been used in several controlled studies to lower blood fats and blood cholesterol. The results of such studies have been inconclusive. Although niacin does lower blood fats and blood cholesterol, it seems to have little effect one way or another in changing the expected rate of future heart attacks or future deaths. The niacinamide form of the vitamin does not lower blood fats by a significant amount.

Niacin is a vasodilator. It may improve circulation in the elderly and thus help keep arms and legs from falling asleep. The overall effectiveness of such a use is unknown, and it may vary from person to person.

Niacin has been used to raise blood sugar levels in cases of hypoglycemia or low blood sugar, reduce high blood pressure, relieve diarrhea, improve circulation, improve digestion, and treat acne.

Reported Side Effects And Unsafe Doses: Niacin has a rather alarming side effect of making the skin flush or turn red. Taking doses of niacin as small as 100 mg., particularly on an empty stomach, can cause flushing, itching and hot feelings especially around the face and neck. This may last for as long as two hours. Flushing is more pronounced in people with blue eyes and in people who have first started to take large doses. Flushing usually disappears or is greatly reduced after large doses have been taken for a few days. The flushing effect from taking niacin may cause a drop in blood pressure. Caution! Niacin should not be used if drugs for treatment of high blood pressure are being taken. A drop in blood pressure may cause dizziness and fainting after getting up from a sitting or lying down position. The flushing effect is absent when the niacinamide form of the vitamin is taken. The niacinamide form of the vitamin may cause mental depression when taken in high doses.

High doses of niacin are reported to cause serious side effects including liver damage, low blood pressure, stomach ulcers, high levels of blood sugar, high levels of uric acid which may lead to gout, dark skin, skin rashes, excitement, irregular heartbeat or skipped heartbeats, heartburn, nausea, vomiting, diarrhea, poor running times in competitive racers.

Large doses of niacin should be avoided by people with poor liver function, past or presently active stomach ulcers, low blood pressure or bleeding problems. Large doses of niacin may also aggravate glaucoma or increase the chances of getting cataracts. Some niacin supplements contain tartrazine as an additive. Tartrazine may cause allergic reactions in some people, especially in people who are allergic to aspirin. Caution! Because niacin is a strong acid and a vasodilator or blood vessel enlarger, it should never be taken on an empty stomach. It should always be taken with food and drink or with a large glass of water and a buffering agent such as the mineral, dolomite, or an antacid preparation.

Pantothenic Acid (Vitamin B5; Calcium Pantothenate)

What It Does: Helps the body use and release energy from carbohydrates . . . necessary for the body to make and break down fatty acids and steroid hormones . . . necessary for normal growth . . . necessary in the functioning of the adrenal glands . . . necessary in antibody production and thus helps combat infection . . . helps the function of the digestive system.

Food Sources: Yeast, whole-grain products, liver, salmon, eggs, beans, seeds, peanuts, mushrooms, elderberries, citrus fruit.

How Long It Stays In Your Body: Pantothenic acid is water soluble, and the body will eliminate much of its store within a few days after withdrawal of pantothenic acid from the diet. Although some pantothenic acid may be made by micro-organisms in the intestines, deficiency symptoms have been reported as soon as two weeks after removal of pantothenic acid from the diet.

Deficiency Diseases And Symptoms: There is no disease specifically associated with a deficiency of pantothenic acid. However, individuals on a diet low in pantothenic acid experience loss of appetite, constipation, low blood pressure, upset stomach, low blood sugar, respiratory infection, burning sensations in the feet, muscle cramps, weakness, fatigue, mood changes, dizziness, psychoses and unsteady walking.

What Reduces, Destroys Or Increases It: Alcohol and caffeine reduce the action of pantothenic acid. Toasting and cooking food destroy much pantothenic acid. Methylbromide, an insecticide used in grain storage

77

areas, destroys some pantothenic acid in the grain.

Recommended Daily Dietary Allowance (RDA): No RDA has been established for pantothenic acid, but the following estimates have been made by the Food and Nutrition Board. Infants 6 mg. - 8 mg.; children 9 mg. - 16 mg.; adult males 16 mg. - 18 mg.; adult females 13 mg. - 15 mg.; pregnant women 15 mg. - 17 mg.; nursing mothers 18 mg. - 20 mg.

Claimed Benefits Of Taking Supplements: Some arthritis sufferers claim that pantothenic acid is effective in reducing pain. A number of British physicians think that pantothenic acid supplements can prevent the development of rheumatoid arthritis and even osteoarthritis in many people. Long-term, controlled studies will be necessary to verify this claim. Pantothenic acid has been reported to reduce unwanted side effects of taking antibiotics. Pantothenic acid supplements may improve stamina and increase life span in animals . . . improve symptoms of senility and depression when taken with other B vitamins . . . lower the incidence of teeth grinding during sleep (bruxism).

Studies have shown that pantothenic acid can be useful following surgery to treat paralytic ileus. Paralytic ileus is a condition which frequently occurs after surgery when intestinal activity stops, causing pain and nausea. Stress, hypoglycemia (low blood sugar), adrenal exhaustion, and infection may be helped by pantothenic acid.

Reported Side Effects And Unsafe Doses: Doses of up to 100 mg. per day have few reported side effects other than diarrhea. Caution! Pantothenic acid may change the action of anticoagulants or antihypertensive drugs.

Cigarette smokers who take pantothenic acid may experience more premature skin wrinkling than smoking causes by itself.

Pyridoxine (Vitamin B6; Pyridoxal Pyridoxamine)

What It Does: Helps the body use protein, carbohydrate and fat ... helps convert the amino acid, tryptophan, which is found in many proteins, to the vitamin niacin or the nervous system hormone, serotonin ... activates numerous enzymes in the body ... helps vitamin B12 absorption into the body ... helps in the production of hydrochloric acid, adrenalin and insulin by the body ... helps regulate fluid levels ... relieves some deficiency symptoms of niacin or riboflavin ... helps the immune system function ... helps produce antibodies and red blood cells.

Food Sources: Yeast, liver, whole-grain products, meat, navy beans, fish, nuts.

How Long It Stays In The Body: Pyridoxine is water soluble. The body can't store it for a long period. Extra amounts which are taken beyond the body's requirements are excreted by the kidneys into the urine after a few hours.

Deficiency Diseases And Symptoms: Pyridoxine deficiency symptoms are similar to the milder deficiency symptoms for niacin or riboflavin. Mild deficiencies of pyridoxine may go undetected, because the only symptoms may be psychological ... depression, lack of dream recall, fatigue or nervousness. Mild deficiencies of pyridoxine may contribute to anemia, hair loss, slow learning, edema or fluid retention during pregnancy and visual disturbances. Mucous membranes around the mouth and lips may become irritated, sore and crack open. Numbness or other changes in feeling may occur. Red blood cell production may be low and cause anemia. Infants with pyridoxine deficiencies may have convulsions. Deficiencies in expectant mothers during the prenatal period may contribute to blood disorders and mental retardation in infants.

What Reduces, Destroys Or Increases It: Oral contraceptives, penicillamine, isoniazid, hydralazine, cortisone, alcohol, caffeine and nicotine can reduce the amount of vitamin B6 in the body. Pyridoxine reduces the effectiveness of barbiturate drugs, levodopa and phenytoin (trade name Dilantin®). Pyridoxine works with other B vitamins and magnesium for maximum effect in the body.

Recommended Daily Dietary Allowance (RDA): Infants 0.3 mg. - 0.6 mg.; children 0.9 mg. - 1.6 mg.; adult males 1.2 mg. - 2.2. mg.; adult females 1.8 mg. - 2.0 mg.; pregnant women 2.4 mg. - 2.6 mg.; nursing mothers 2.3 mg. - 2.5 mg.

Claimed Benefits Of Taking Supplements: Magnesium oxide and pyridoxine have been used to limit or stop calcium oxalate clumping which is a major cause of kidney stones. Taking supplements of 25 mg. of pyridoxine per day may help prevent kidney stone occurrence or recurrence.

Average levels of pyridoxine are found to be lower for men and women over 50. In women, an increase in estrogen levels (occurring during pregnancy, during the menstrual cycle, and when taking oral contraceptives) increases the body's need for pyridoxine. In women, pyridoxine supplementation may reduce or improve symptoms of depression, pre-menstrual fluid retention and weight gain, pre-menstrual acne and menopausal arthritis. Pyridoxine supplementation may reduce or improve symptoms associated with these conditions.

Toxemia of pregnancy, sometimes called eclampsia, may be helped by pyridoxine late in pregnancy. Pyridoxine may relieve "morning sickness" in the first three months of pregnancy, and it may also relieve motion sickness.

There is a genetic defect which causes homocystinuria, an enzyme deficiency disease. In homocystinuria, byproducts of the body's metabolism build up and cause mental retardation and damage to the arteries. Large doses of pyridoxine can activate the defective enzyme in about half the cases treated with 200 mg. - 500 mg. per day initially, then with lower doses later in the treatment.

Pyridoxine deficiency may contribute to hardening of the arteries and coronary heart disease. Pyridoxine supplementation may be especially helpful in preventing heart and artery disease for people who eat high-protein diets. When meat is cooked, it loses much of its pyridoxine which could have been used by the body to help break down methionine, one of the amino acids found in protein. Byproducts of methionine are thought to damage the arteries and cause heart disease much like the process which is involved to a much greater extent in homocystinuria. Taking small supplements of pyridoxine with each meal containing cooked meat may help to prevent some coronary heart disease.

Taking 25 mg. - 50 mg. of pyridoxine per day may help improve symptoms of carpal tunnel syndrome, a condition where a nerve in the hand is irritated by pressure from the bones and cartilage around it. Reported cases of improvement in carpal tunnel syndrome symptoms have taken place after people had taken pyridoxine supplements for two or more months.

Pyridoxine may relieve symptoms of asthma and reduce

the frequency, duration and severity of asthmatic attacks. Dr. Robert Reynolds, a U. S. Department of Agriculture research chemist, has reported that symptoms "were relieved in every asthmatic tested" when they received 50 mg. of pyridoxine twice a day. Most patients in the study did not notice an improvement in their asthmatic symptoms until they had taken pyridoxine for a period of four weeks.

Pyridoxine may increase energy levels and improve resistance to stress. It has been used to try to help prevent or treat baldness, ulcers, diabetes, and tooth decay.

Reported Side Effects And Unsafe Doses: Taking large doses of pyridoxine can damage the nervous system. Symptoms include loss of sensation in the hands and feet, unsteady walking and numbness around the mouth. Upon examination by a physician, other signs and symptoms have been noted, including loss of reflexes in the arms and legs, loss of position and vibration sense in the outer arms, legs, hands and feet, and loss of sensations detecting pain, temperature, pinprick and touch. Most victims recover partially or completely within several months after they stop taking large doses of the vitamin. The dosage level where nervous system damage has been reported is 500 mg. per day or more, but anyone taking pyridoxine supplements for anything other than severe cases of homocystinuria should take far less than this amount.

The drug Bendectin®, which is reported to cause birth defects, contains pyridoxine. Taking pyridoxine early in pregnancy may contribute to a small increase in certain types of birth defects. Pyridoxine supplementation can prevent milk from flowing in mothers who want to nurse their children. Taking as little as 25 mg. of pyridoxine in the evening is reported to frequently cause vivid dreams or poor sleep. Taking pyridoxine at high dosage levels of 200 mg. per day for 30 days is reported to cause withdrawal symptoms if taking the vitamin is suddenly stopped.

Riboflavin (Vitamin B2)

What It Does: Helps the body's cells use oxygen . . . helps in the growth and maintenance of body tissues . . . helps maintain healthy skin, nails and hair . . . promotes absorption of iron . . . helps vision . . . helps the body use proteins and fats . . . regulates hormones . . . helps to activate vitamin B6.

Food Sources: Yeast, liver and other organ meats, eggs, milk, dairy products, whole-grain products, nuts, leafy green vegetables and mushrooms. White flour often is enriched with riboflavin.

How Long It Stays In Your Body: Riboflavin is a water-soluble vitamin. The body cannot store extra amounts of it, and extra amounts which are taken are usually flushed out through the kidneys. Deficiency symptoms may start to show up within a week after withdrawal of riboflavin from the diet.

Deficiency Diseases And Symptoms: Mild deficiencies of riboflavin may go undetected, because the only symptoms may be psychological . . . depression, fatigue or nervousness. Mild deficiencies of riboflavin may contribute to anemia, oily skin, baldness, dizziness, and sluggishness.

Severe riboflavin deficiency first causes ulcers or pain in the mouth and other mucous membranes. The lips may become pale or red. The tongue becomes sore and purplish in color. Eyes become bloodshot, eyelids become inflamed, and pupils may become dilated. Sensitivity to light may occur. The skin may become red, scaly and greasy as the disease progresses.

What Reduces, Destroys Or Increases It: Riboflavin

is easily destroyed by light. Milk which has been on supermarket shelves in clear containers that light can penetrate loses much of its riboflavin. Antibiotics, oral contraceptives, alcohol and baking soda deplete riboflavin in the body. Regular vigorous exercise, especially in women, may cause riboflavin deficiency. High-protein diets deplete riboflavin. Vitamin A, vitamin E and other B vitamins work together with riboflavin for greatest benefit in the body.

Recommended Daily Dietary Allowance (RDA): Infants 0.4 mg. - 0.6 mg.; children 0.8 mg. - 1.4 mg.; adult males 1.4 mg. - 1.7 mg.; adult females 1.2 mg. - 1.3 mg.; pregnant women 1.5 mg. - 1.6 mg.; nursing mothers 1.7 mg. - 1.8 mg.

Claimed Benefits Of Taking Supplements: Riboflavin deficiency may be one cause of cataracts. Unconfirmed reports of recovery from cataracts have been made when supplements of riboflavin were taken. Although not proven, riboflavin may decrease the damage caused by allergies to the lining of the eye and the damage of other immunological disorders.

Riboflavin in pregnant women may decrease the possibility of birth defects. Laboratory studies indicate that animals who are deficient in riboflavin had high rates of birth defects. Studies have shown that pregnant women who are in a high-risk group for delivering children with birth defects had much lower rates of delivering children with birth defects when they took multivitamins during pregnancy. Extra riboflavin may be needed by people with hyperthyroidism because of the higher energy output of the body.

High protein intake requires high riboflavin intake for proper metabolism. People with illnesses where doctors have advised higher protein intake, such as certain ulcer or diabetic diets, may be lacking enough riboflavin.

Reported Side Effects And Unsafe Doses: Riboflavin, when taken in the absence of other nutritional supplements such as other B vitamins and vitamins C and E, may cause sensitivity to sunlight.

Large doses of riboflavin (50 to 100 mg./day) have been found to reverse symptoms of deficiency as long as permanent damage to the organs originating the symptoms has not occurred.

Excesses are excreted by the kidneys once tissues are saturated with high doses of riboflavin. If side effects occur, they are generally mild and short term, since riboflavin is not stored by the body. Nausea is the most common side effect when levels become too high. Sensitivity or allergy to riboflavin preparations may be a danger for some people.

Thiamine (Vitamin B1)

What It Does: Thiamine is essential for the body to use carbohydrates for its energy requirements. It's needed for the growth and repair of body tissues . . . transmission of nerve impulses . . . maintenance of muscle tone and movement within the stomach and intestines . . . important for learning, intelligence, mental attitude and good appetite.

Food Sources: Yeast, liver, whole-grain products, wheat, eggs, milk, nuts, potatoes, leafy green vegetables, kidney beans and seeds are good natural sources of thiamine. Most white flour and some white rice are enriched with thiamine.

How Long It Stays In Your Body: Thiamine is water soluble and body tissues cannot store it for long. It is used up quickly by the body. Deficiency symptoms may occur within five days of withdrawal of thiamine from the diet. Excesses of thiamine are excreted by the kidneys, reducing the danger of buildup of this vitamin to harmful levels in the body.

Deficiency Diseases And Symptoms: Beri-beri, a disease which affects the nervous system and the circulatory system, is caused by thiamine deficiency. Early symptoms include fatigue, weight loss, loss of appetite, irritability, sleep disturbances, memory loss, poor concentration, depression, abdominal discomfort, constipation, muscle weakness, cramps, chest pain, and loss of feeling with tingling or burning sensations. Prolonged deficiencies may lead to mental confusion, poor reflexes eventually leading to paralysis, fluid retention leading to swelling of hands and feet, and poor heart function.

Thiamine deficiency may also be caused by intestinal illnesses such as chronic diarrhea which interfere with absorption into the body. Severe liver disease can cause symptoms of thiamine deficiency.

What Reduces, Destroys Or Increases It: Inadequate dietary intake is the main cause of thiamine deficiency. Steaming or exposure to moist heat greatly reduces the thiamine content of food. Soaking vegetables or toasting bread or other baked goods reduces thiamine content. Some uncooked seafood, such as clams, contain an enzyme which can destroy thiamine. Complete milling of grain to produce white rice or white flour removes the bran and the germ which contain most of the thiamine found in grain.

The need for thiamine is increased when carbohydrate consumption is high. Exercise or emotional stress may increase the energy needs of the body and the body's need for thiamine. More thiamine is needed in pregnancy, during breastfeeding, when fever is present, during and after surgery, and in cases of hyperthyroidism.

Sulfa drugs and other antibiotics may deplete thiamine. Estrogens such as those found in oral contraceptives create deficiencies. Air pollution and food additives (especially nitrates and sulfates) may increase the body's need for thiamine.

Other B vitamins, vitamin C, vitamin E, growth hormone, manganese and magnesium may increase the activity of thiamine in the body. Vitamins C and E, and growth hormone (STH), also increase the positive effects of thiamine. Manganese and magnesium play a role in activating enzymes requiring thiamine and increase the effectiveness of thiamine.

The intestinal tract provides the acid surroundings needed for absorption of thiamine. Substances which change the acid level, making it too alkaline (even common baking soda) or extremely acid, can interfere with the absorption of thiamine.

B vitamins complement each other. A balance is needed of B1, B2, B3, B6, B12, folic acid, biotin, and pantothenic acid for the most efficient utilization.

Recommended Daily Dietary Allowances (RDA):
Infants 0.3 mg. - 0.5 mg.; children 0.7 mg. - 1.2 mg.; adult males 1.2 mg. - 1.5 mg.; adult females 1.0 mg. - 1.1 mg.; pregnant females 1.4 mg. - 1.5 mg.; nursing mothers 1.5 mg. - 1.6 mg.

Claimed Benefits Of Taking Supplements: Today's nutritional habits may produce mild deficiencies. More thiamine-deficient, refined sugars and starches are eaten. Thiamine is essential for proper metabolism of carbohydrates. More carbohydrates in the diet require more thiamine to be present to break them down.

Heart patients who have a higher intake of processed carbohydrates have been found to have lower levels of thiamine in the body. Thiamine is needed for muscle tone and in order for energy to be supplied to the heart muscle.

Aging may be a reason for taking supplemental thiamine. Changes in taste, financial changes which alter dietary intake, and normal changes in the intestinal lining with aging can result in a decrease of thiamine levels.

Some studies suggest that higher thiamine intake may improve mental abilities for some people.

Alcoholics can benefit from thiamine supplements. Alcohol is a carbohydrate equivalent, and the body requires extra thiamine to break it down and use it. Regular, heavy consumption of alcohol is accompanied by a decrease in food intake and vitamins. Alcoholism causes liver damage which reduces the body's ability to use thiamine efficiently. Thiamine and other vitamin supplements may decrease alcohol dependence in alcoholics. Thiamine supplements may reduce some of the damage that smoking and alcoholism do to the body. Because of rapid excretion through the kidneys, alcoholics and others who take large doses of B vitamins usually take them in three or four equal portions during the day to maintain constant high levels in the blood.

Large doses of thiamine taken by mouth or by injection (50 to 100 mg./day) have been found to reverse symptoms of deficiency as long as permanent damage to the organs in which the symptoms originated has not occurred.

Reported Side Effects And Unsafe Doses: Few side effects except for nausea and allergic reactions have been reported after taking high doses of thiamine. Excesses are excreted by the kidneys once tissues are saturated with thiamine. If side effects occur, they are generally mild and short term, since thiamine is not stored by the body. Nausea is the most common side effect when levels become too high. Sensitivity or allergy to thiamine preparations may be a danger for some people.

People with diabetes mellitus (sugar diabetes) should consult their physicians before taking thiamine supplements, because large doses may inactivate insulin.

Large doses of a single B vitamin can result in artificial deficiencies of other B vitamins. B6 may be significantly reduced by an oversupply of thiamine. Taking equal amounts of the following B vitamins: thiamine, riboflavin, niacin, pyridoxine and pantothenic acid has been suggested as a way to avoid artificial deficiencies.

Thiamine may protect smokers and drinkers from some of the damage that they do to their bodies.

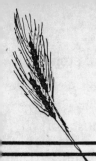

Minerals

Calcium

What It Does: Essential for the functioning of the nervous and muscular systems . . . essential for blood clotting and heart function . . . essential for bone growth . . . strengthens cell walls and membranes. Calcium is also reported to act as a mild tranquilizer.

Food Sources: Dairy products are the richest sources of calcium. Other sources are leafy, green vegetables, salmon, sardines and calcium present in the water supply. Other foods may contain small amounts of calcium.

How Long It Stays In Your Body: Many years' supply of calcium is stored in the body's bones, and the body can use this store to supply calcium for essential functions.

Deficiency Diseases And Symptoms: Low levels of calcium in the blood may cause muscle cramps, pounding heartbeat, loss of sleep and tooth decay. Long-term calcium deficiency may cause osteoporosis, osteomalacia or rickets, diseases which involve the loss of calcium from the bones or the failure of the growing bones to have enough calcium for strength and proper growth.

What Reduces, Destroys Or Increases It: Excessive consumption of phosphorus, as found in most soft drinks, drives calcium out of the bones and leads to osteoporosis. Excessive consumption of protein, as found in the typical American diet, also leads to a loss of calcium. Vitamin D increases the absorption of calcium. Oral contraceptives and the female hormone estrogen increase the absorption of calcium into the body. Vitamin D promotes the absorption and retention of calcium.

Substances found in food including oxalic acid (found in rhubarb and spinach), phosphorus (found in soft drinks and in many other foods), phytic acid (found in whole-grain products) and corticosteroid drugs, such as cortisone, interfere with calcium absorption or cause the body to lose calcium. Tobacco, alcohol and caffeine may interfere with the absorption of calcium or the body's ability to retain calcium.

Lack of exercise, high-fluoride intake, emotional stress, prolonged bed rest, pregnancy, menopause, and high temperatures are conditions which require an increased intake of calcium.

Recommended Daily Dietary Allowance (RDA): Infants 360 - 540 mg.; children 800 mg.; adult males 800 - 1200 mg.; adult females 800 -1200 mg.; pregnant women 1200 - 1600 mg.; nursing mothers 1200 - 1600 mg.

Claimed Benefits Of Taking Supplements: Nutritional authorities agree that most adult Americans do not consume the RDA of calcium. Many nutritional authorities suggest that moderate calcium, estrogen and possibly vitamin D supplementation can help prevent osteoporosis in aging women and also in aging men (minus estrogen).

Osteoporosis causes the collapse of the backbone in many elderly people and contributes to hip fractures which are especially likely in the elderly.

Calcium supplements may help to lower many cases of high blood pressure. Adequate calcium is necessary during periods of rapid bone growth in childhood and during pregnancy and nursing. Calcium supplements are used to treat tetany, or muscle contractions in newborn infants, muscle cramps, bone pain, and low parathyroid function and conditions which mimic it.

Reported Side Effects And Unsafe Doses: Calcium supplementation should be avoided by people who have kidney stones or by people who have high blood levels of calcium which may favor the formation of kidney stones. Calcium supplements should not be taken within one hour of taking tetracycline antibiotic drugs, because calcium may reduce blood levels of these antibiotics. Calcium supplements interfere with the action of verapamil, a calcium-channel blocker used in the treatment of heart disease patients.

Symptoms of calcium overdose include loss of appetite, nausea, vomiting, constipation, abdominal pain, dryness of the mouth, thirst and frequent urination. High blood levels of calcium can cause fatalities in premature infants. Taking large amounts of calcium, especially if calcium is taken with vitamin D, can lead to the deposit of calcium in many soft tissues of the body, such as the walls of the arteries and the kidneys. Taking calcium supplements in the form of bone meal can lead to the excessive consumption of lead, a poisonous metal. Most bone meal contains high levels of lead which is concentrated in bones in the food chain. Taking calcium supplements in the form of dolomite, a mineral containing calcium carbonate and magnesium carbonate, may, in some cases, lead to the accumulation of lead in the body. Most large companies which sell dolomite have taken steps to see that their supplies are low in lead. Other smaller companies are in the process of "getting the lead out."

Chromium

What It Does: Helps the body use carbohydrates efficiently . . . helps the action of insulin . . . evens out high or low swings in blood sugar levels.

Food Sources: Brewer's yeast, mushrooms, corn, meat, cheese and whole grains are good sources of chromium.

How Long It Stays In Your Body: Unknown.

Deficiency Diseases And Symptoms: Poor glucose metabolism (sugar use) and the aggravation of diabetes are deficiency symptoms.

What Reduces, Destroys Or Increases It: Unknown.

Recommended Daily Dietary Allowance (RDA): Infants 10 - 60 microgram§ (mcg.); children 20 - 200 mcg.; adults 50 - 200 mcg.

Claimed Benefits Of Taking Supplements: Studies have shown that chromium supplements can even out swings in blood sugar levels in people who have a tendency toward low blood sugar (hypoglycemia) or high blood sugar (hyperglycemia). Chromium supplements may aid in the treatment of maturity-onset diabetes and problems which are associated with diabetes, such as a tendency toward infections, heart and circulatory problems. To the extent that chromium may help regulate blood sugar levels and overeating which may lead to being overweight, chromium may help reduce the incidence of some kinds of cancer.

Reported Side Effects And Unsafe Doses: Safety levels for chromium have not been established, but safety levels for other trace elements like chromium are usually not far above the recommended levels.

Copper

What It Does: Helps in the formation of bone, hair and skin . . . important in the formation of hemoglobin and red blood cells . . . helps the healing processes of the body.

Food Sources: Liver and organ meats, seafood, oranges, eggs, green leafy vegetables, raisins, nuts and legumes are rich sources of copper.

How Long It Stays In Your Body: Unknown. It is suspected that the body has mechanisms for maintaining enough copper for several weeks before obvious deficiency symptoms occur.

Deficiency Diseases And Symptoms: Anemia, bone disease, blood cell abnormalities, degeneration of the nervous system, defects in the pigmentation and structure of hair, failure of the reproductive system, damage to the heart and arteries.

What Reduces, Destroys Or Increases It: High intake of zinc and high intake of vitamin C reduce copper or interfere with some of its actions. High amounts of molybdenum in the diet or in the water interfere with the absorption and utilization of copper. Oral contraceptives reduce the need for copper.

Recommended Daily Dietary Allowance (RDA): Infants .5 mg. - 1 mg.; children 1 mg. - 2.5 mg.; adults 2 mg. - 3 mg.

Claimed Benefits Of Taking Supplements: People who take large doses of vitamin C or zinc can become anemic, because these nutrients interfere with the body's use of copper which is important in the formation of red blood cells.

Reported Side Effects And Unsafe Doses: Copper can be poisonous in doses several times higher than the RDA. Copper, even in small doses, can accumulate in and damage the livers of people like alcoholics who have poor liver function.

Fluoride (Fluorine)

What It Does: Helps prevent cavities.

Food Sources: Fluoride is found in the soil and water in certain areas of the country. People who live in areas of high-fluoride concentration consume more fluoride than people living in areas of low-fluoride concentration. Food grown or processed in areas of high natural fluoride concentration, or in areas with fluoridated water supplies, often is transported to other areas. This helps even out geographical differences in fluoride intake.

How Long It Stays In Your Body: Fluoride remains in the body for a long time; because it is incorporated into the bones.

Deficiency Diseases And Symptoms: There is no deficiency disease.

What Reduces, Destroys Or Increases It: Fluoride is added to many water supplies and to food processed in areas containing high levels of fluoride. Fluoride may be added to the soil in certain fertilizers. Fluoride is added to most toothpaste. It is also found in seafood, garlic, and oats.

Recommended Daily Dietary Allowance (RDA): Infants .10 - 1 mg.; children 0.5 - 2.5 mg.; adults 1.5 mg. - 4 mg.

Claimed Benefits Of Taking Supplements: Stronger tooth enamel and bones . . . fewer cavities . . . fewer bone fractures . . . less osteoporosis in older women . . . higher birth weights and higher rates of growth in children . . . reduced loss of hearing if caused by otospongeosis of the inner ear.

Reported Side Effects And Unsafe Doses: The addition of fluoride to water supplies has been a controversial issue in the United States for many years. A majority of the members of the scientific, medical and dental professions support the addition of fluoride to water supplies. A minority of researchers, however, point out the proven harmful effects of taking just a little more than the recommended levels of fluoride. They question whether all of these effects are absent at the recommended levels.

The damage done by fluoride is increased in people on low protein diets. The higher the dose of fluoride, the greater the chance of side effects. The following side effects have been reported at doses within or above the RDA: painful and aching bones, stiffness, weakness, chalky white areas on the teeth (mild overdose), brown or pitted teeth (severe overdose), knots on the bones (exostoses), rapid aging, increased rates of cancer, high death rate (up to three times higher in areas of high fluoride concentration in the water supply), sagging and wrinkled skin, scleroderma (hard patches of skin), loss of calcium from the bones leading to osteoporosis or osteomalacia (reports of this last side effect contradict other reports that small doses of fluoride may be helpful in strengthening bones).

People in India sometimes suffer from the bone deformities (i.e. hunchback) of skeletal fluorosis even when the fluoride concentration in the water is only one and one half times the RDA! Hot weather, drinking lots of water and low protein diets increase fluoride intake and side effects.

The use of fluoridated water in kidney dialysis machines often causes severe side effects or fatalities. Large doses of fluoride are extremely poisonous. The death rate in

Annapolis, Md. increased to three times normal after the local water system accidentally added too much to their fluoridated water supply. Sudden death in infants may occur with the consumption of five to ten times the recommended level. People living in warm areas in the United States or people who exercise a lot may consume too much fluoride if they drink lots of fluoridated water or other fluids such as reconstituted juice made with fluoridated water. A table prepared by the Centers for Disease Control says that people living in the hottest areas of the United States consume almost twice as much fluoride on the average as people living in the coldest areas of the United States.

Fluoride may cause increased rates of cancer. This reported side effect is the subject of much debate. Some studies show a link between higher rates of cancer and the fluoridation of water supplies. Other studies show little or no link. People on both sides of this debate have correctly accused each other of using wrong methodology and making errors in their scientific studies.

Author's Opinion: The addition of fluoride to water supplies has been promoted as an effective way to reduce dental decay in children, and it has been proven to be effective for this purpose. Once permanent teeth come in, fluoride has little or no effect in preventing decay. Excessive fluoride in the diet and in the water supply has many proven bad side effects. The greater the amount of fluoride in the diet or in the water, the more likely it is that serious side effects will occur.

Fluoride is widely available in toothpaste. A recent inspection of a local supermarket shelf revealed eight brands of toothpaste which contained fluoride and only two brands which did not contain fluoride. If people want to make sure their children receive a fluoride supplement so they will have fewer cavities, all they have to do is to use a fluoride toothpaste. Caution: Small children often swallow large amounts of toothpaste. Be careful of overdoses in them.

Some dental authorities argue that low-fluoride water supplies should be fluoridated, because fluoride in food and water is more effective in preventing decay in children than fluoride toothpaste. However, much fluoride gets into the diet even in areas where it's low in the water. Small amounts of fluoride toothpaste are usually swallowed inadvertently after brushing, and foods pick up extra fluoride from fertilizers and from processing in areas with fluoridated water supplies. In a recent study, people in Salt Lake City had higher than recommended levels of fluoride in their bodies even though their water supply is low in fluoride. Many people in areas where the water supply is fluoridated receive much more than the recommended levels.

Since fluoride is widely available on a selective basis to anyone who wants to use it, it seems to me to be a questionable health practice to add a possibly harmful substance to the water or to the diet of everyone. Anyone who is concerned about possible side effects from fluoride overdose, if the local water supply is fluoridated or high in natural fluorides, should drink fruit juice, not prepared from concentrate, produced in areas of low-fluoride concentration such as most apple growing regions or use water bottled in regions of low fluoride concentration. (My personal preference is Mountain Valley Water. It's low in sodium, and it has a good balance of necessary minerals.)

Iodine (Iodide)

What It Does: Helps form thyroid hormone which affects the body's production of energy and mental and physical development.

Food Sources: Shellfish, seafood, kelp, garlic, pears, pineapple, and mushrooms contain iodine. Amounts in most other sources depend on the amounts of iodine in the soil.

How Long It Stays In Your Body: Iodine is concentrated in the thyroid gland. If stores in the gland are adequate, the body can retain enough for its use for several months or even for years.

Deficiency Diseases And Symptoms: Symptoms of deficiency are related to the symptoms of hypothyroidism (low production of thyroid hormone). Symptoms may include tiredness, irritability, obesity, cold hands and feet, heart palpitations, nervousness, dry hair and skin and goiter (a noticeable enlargement of the thyroid gland in the neck). In infants and children mental retardation may occur. Iodine is routinely added to table salt in the United States, and deficiency symptoms in this country are rare.

What Reduces, Destroys Or Increases It: Unknown.

Recommended Daily Dietary Allowance (RDA): Infants 40 - 50 <u>micrograms</u> (<u>mcg</u>.); children 70 -120 <u>mcg</u>.; adult males 150 <u>mcg</u>.; adult females 150 <u>mcg</u>.; pregnant women 175 <u>mcg</u>.; nursing mothers 200 <u>mcg</u>.

Claimed Benefits Of Taking Supplements: The avoidance of goiter or hypothyroidism in areas where there is little iodine in the soil.

Reported Side Effects And Unsafe Doses: Harmful levels for many trace elements, including iodine, may be only a few times the RDA; so the RDA should not be greatly exceeded.

Iron

What It Does: Essential for the formation of hemoglobin, myoglobin and many enzymes . . . necessary for the formation of red blood cells which help carry oxygen to the body and help fight stress and disease.

Food Sources: Whole-grain products, liver and organ meats, red meat, eggs, lima beans, prunes, spinach, raw broccoli, peas, fish and raisins are all good sources.

How Long It Stays İn Your Body: Iron is stored in the body in the form of ferritin in the body's bone marrow and organs. Low red blood cell counts in laboratory tests may not show up for many months after iron has become deficient in the diet.

Deficiency Diseases And Symptoms: Slight iron deficiency which do not affect red blood cell counts may cause tiredness, headache, slower running times in competitive runners, irritability or depression and sleeplessness or troubled sleep. Severe iron deficiency may cause anemia or low red blood cell counts, constipation, mouth soreness, brittle nails, pale skin or difficulty in breathing.

What Reduces, Destroys Or Increases It: Vitamin E and zinc taken in large doses interfere with the absorption of iron. Caffeine from coffee, tea or soft drinks interferes with the absorption of iron. Excessive phosphorus consumption in people who eat lots of canned food or in people who drink many soft drinks may block iron absorption. Excessive sweating can eliminate extra iron from the body. Rapid food transit time through the intestines in people who eat high-fiber diets can reduce the absorption of iron. Foot pounding in runners can destroy red blood cells and cause iron to be eliminated from the body. Excessive bleeding as in women who have heavy menstrual periods increases the loss of iron from the body. Women who use intrauterine devices (IUDs) lose more blood than normal in menstrual bleeding. Women who use oral contraceptives lose less blood than normal because they bleed less.

Cooking food in cast-iron pots and pans adds to the diet. This has been recommended as a good way of getting a moderate amount of supplemental iron.

Other factors which increase the need for iron include any blood loss, hemorrhoids, peptic ulcers, and colitis.

Recommended Daily Dietary Allowance (RDA): Infants 10 - 15 mg.; children 10 - 15 mg.; adult males 10 - 18 mg.; adult females 10 - 18 mg.; pregnant women 40 - 78 mg.; nursing mothers 40 - 78 mg for first 3 months, then 10-18 mg. Note: The Recommended Daily Dietary Allowance of iron for pregnant women and newly nursing mothers cannot be met by ordinary diet Therefore, the use of supplemental iron is recommended during pregnancy and for two or three months after giving birth, at which point normal RDAs for adult females should be resumed.

Claimed Benefits Of Taking Supplements: Taking extra iron is recommended by the United States Government during pregnancy and breast feeding. Many women, especially those who have heavy menstrual flow, can benefit from taking extra iron. People who are fatigued may sometimes benefit from taking extra iron. Runners, people who work or exercise heavily in hot temperatures and people who eat high-fiber food may benefit from taking extra iron. Benefits include increased stamina and protection against anemia.

Reported Side Effects And Unsafe Doses: Unlike most other vitamins and minerals, iron is not automatically thrown off by the body, but is stored. Therefore, taking too much iron can cause unhealthy iron deposits in the body. Anyone with iron-storage disease, in which excessive amounts of iron are deposited in the body, should be very cautious about taking iron supplements.

Since iron is stored and not thrown off by the body, any supplements of iron should closely parallel the recommended daily allowances after adjustment has been made for the amount of iron in the diet.

Iron supplements interfere with the absorption of antibiotics like tetracycline. Iron supplements deactivate vitamin E and vitamin C.

Accidental overdoses of iron can cause bleeding from the stomach or intestines and a drop in blood pressure. Fatalities have occurred in children who have swallowed their mothers' iron supplements. Excessive amounts of iron in the bloodstream provide an environment which helps bacteria, viruses and fungi grow. Too much iron may cause reduced resistance to infections. Iron, even in small doses, can accumulate in and damage the livers of people like alcoholics who have poor liver function.

Magnesium

What It Does: Magnesium works with calcium in a number of ways. It's used with calcium and phosphorus in the formation of bone. It's important in many enzyme systems and in maintaining electrical potential in nerves and muscles. It is used in carbohydrate and mineral metabolism.

Food Sources: Magnesium is widely distributed in water and in many other foods. Whole-grain products, vegetables, black-eyed peas, bananas, apples, peaches, lima beans, seafood and peanuts are good sources of magnesium. The water supply is also an excellent source of magnesium in many areas of the country where the water is relatively hard.

How Long It Stays In Your Body: Even though magnesium is stored in the bone, it is important to have regular intake to maintain magnesium concentrations in the body's fluids.

Deficiency Diseases And Symptoms: Muscle tremors and convulsions, especially in infants and children, nervousness, irritability, leg cramps, and excessive excitability are deficiency symptoms. A severe magnesium deficiency may result in coronary heart disease, mental confusion, and blood clot formation.

What Reduces, Destroys Or Increases It: Alcohol, diuretics, emotional or physical stress, diarrhea, zinc, and fluoride increase the need for magnesium.

Recommended Daily Dietary Allowance (RDA): Infants 50 - 70 mg.; children 150 - 250 mg.; adult males 350 - 400 mg.; adult females 300 mg.; pregnant women 450 mg.; nursing mothers 450 mg.

Claimed Benefits Of Taking Supplements: Proper heart function and the avoidance of heart attacks which are related to electrolyte imbalances, lower rates of depression, kidney stones, nervousness and stomach acidity.

Magnesium and vitamin B6 have been used successfully in controlled scientific studies to greatly reduce the reoccurrence of calcium oxalate kidney stones. Magnesium may help combat stress, maintain muscle contractions, and may aid in adaptation to cold.

Reported Side Effects And Unsafe Doses: If people have normal kidney function, there is little reported danger from overdose. 3 - 5 g. of magnesium taken per day may cause diarrhea or excessive bowel movements in some people; however, small amounts of magnesium are reported to be constipating.

Manganese

What It Does: Helps fertility and reproduction . . . helps growth and sex hormone production . . . helps form bone and cartilage . . . helps regulate blood sugar . . . helps the body use proteins and carbohydrates.

Food Sources: Whole-grain products, fruits (especially bananas), vegetables (especially legumes), liver and other organ meats and eggs.

How Long It Stays In Your Body: Manganese is not known to be stored in any special way, so it's assumed that regular dietary manganese is desirable.

Deficiency Diseases And Symptoms: Poor fertility, miscarriages, poor growth rates in children, birth defects, poor growth of bone and cartilage, poor muscle co-ordination, dizziness, ringing in the ears and other hearing problems and high levels of blood sugar have been reported as symptoms of manganese deficiency.

What Reduces, Destroys Or Increases It: Excessive intake of calcium or phosphorus may reduce the availability of manganese.

Recommended Daily Dietary Allowance (RDA): Infants 0.5 - 1.0 mg.; children up to age six 1.0 - 2.0 mg.; children over age six 2.0 - 5.0 mg.; adults 2.5 - 5.0 mg.

Claimed Benefits Of Taking Supplements: Reduction in allergic reactions in cases of asthma . . : improvement in some cases of diabetes . . . reduced tiredness . . . improved muscle co-ordination.

Reported Side Effects and Unsafe Doses: Manganese

is known to be highly toxic when inhaled or when taken intravenously, but it is much less toxic when taken as a dietary supplement in large doses. Nevertheless, as with all trace minerals, it is best to stay close to the RDA.

Phosphorus

What It Does: Along with calcium, provides much of the structure of bone . . . helps in bone and tooth formation, cell growth, nerve and muscle activity and energy transfer metabolism . . . activates many of the B vitamins . . . is present in blood and body cells as well as in fats, proteins and carbohydrates.

Food Sources: Phosphorus is present in nearly all foods, especially soft drinks, and high protein foods such as meat, fish, whole grains, eggs, dried fruits, and corn. Dietary deficiency is extremely unlikely to occur. As a matter of fact, the main problem with phosphorus in the modern American diet is too much, not too little.

How Long It Stays In Your Body Phosphorus is present in the bone. The body can draw upon this store in emergencies.

Deficiency Diseases And Symptoms: Phosphorus deficiency can occur as a result of prolonged and excessive intake of non-absorbable antacids, like mineral oil. Symptoms are weakness, loss of appetite, "unwell feeling", and pain in the bones.

What Reduces, Destroys Or Increases It: High consumption of soft drinks, canned and other processed foods introduces excessive amounts of phosphorus into the body.

Recommended Daily Dietary Allowance (RDA): Infants 240 - 360 mg.; children 800 mg.; adult males 800 - 1200 mg.; adult females 800 - 1200 mg.; pregnant women 1200 - 1600 mg.; nursing mothers 1200 - 1600 mg.

Claimed Benefits Of Taking Supplements: Claimed benefits of taking phosphorus supplements are related to the reduction in deficiency symptoms which are rare.

Reported Side Effects And Unsafe Doses: Taking more than the RDA of phosphorus may drive calcium out of the bones. Excessive phosphorus in the diet contributes to osteoporosis, or the loss of calcium from the bones, which is found in older people, especially in older women. Excessive phosphorus in the diet can aggravate other conditions which may cause the loss of calcium from the bones. The best ratios of calcium to phosphorus in the diet range from 2 parts calcium to 1 part phosphorus up to 1 part phosphorus to 1 part calcium. Reducing consumption of soft drinks and meat is helpful in reducing phosphorus intake.

Potassium

What It Does: Serves as an essential electrolyte in the body by helping to transmit electro-chemical impulses . . . important for chemical reactions within the body's cells and the regulation of nervous system and muscle system function . . . plays a part in the regulation of blood pressure.

Food Sources: Potassium is widely distributed in most foods. Meat, potatoes, raisins, nuts, tomatoes, bananas, milk and fruit are good sources.

How Long It Stays In The Body: The body can conserve potassium when intake is low by excreting less through the kidneys into the urine. Deficiency symptoms in adults usually don't appear until intake is in the lower range of the RDA for infants.

Deficiency Diseases And Symptoms: Insomnia, dry skin, irregular heartbeat, weakness, poor muscle function, poor reflexes, irritability, thirst and constipation are possible symptoms of low levels of potassium.

What Reduces, Destroys Or Increases It: Prescription drugs, especially some diuretics, can cause excessive potassium loss from the body. Kidney problems can cause potassium to build up to high levels in the body. Diarrhea, diabetic acidosis and certain laxatives can cause excessive loss of potassium.

Recommended Daily Dietary Allowance (RDA): Infants 350 -1275 mg.; children 550 - 3000 mg.; adults 1525 - 5625 mg.

Claimed Benefits Of Taking Supplements: Reduction

in high blood pressure, lower rates of heart disease and heart attack, less fluid retention.

Reported Side Effects And Unsafe Doses: People with kidney problems and people taking potassium-sparing diuretics should avoid taking extra potassium, because it may build up to high levels in the body.

Poisonous levels for most adults may be reached by taking 18 grams per day, or more than three times the maximum recommended daily allowance. Fatalities may result when high levels of potassium in the bloodstream cause heart attacks. It is strongly recommended that the rather high recommended daily allowance for potassium not be exceeded. The body is capable of conserving potassium at times when dietary intake is low.

Selenium

What It Does: Selenium is a co-factor in an enzyme which protects body tissues, especially cell membranes, from oxidation by unstable free radicals. Free radicals can be produced naturally in the body or by pollution or radiation.

Food Sources: Liver and other organ meats, seafood, eggs, onions, meat, poultry, grains, cereals, dairy products and vegetables. Grain products grown in Colorado, New Mexico, Montana, Wyoming, North Dakota, South Dakota and certain other areas may have higher concentrations of selenium than grains grown in other areas of the country where selenium levels in the soil are low.

How Long It Stays In Your Body: Unknown.

Deficiency Diseases And Symptoms: In China, where food is not widely distributed across the country but is grown and consumed largely in the same area, heart muscle abnormalities have been reported in children in areas of the country which are low in selenium. Animals fed a selenium-free diet suffer from degeneration of muscles and liver. A selenium deficiency may result in symptoms of premature aging.

What Reduces, Destroys Or Increases It: The refining of flour removes much of the selenium which is concentrated in the germ and bran. Therefore, it is important to eat whole-grain products since selenium is not added back into enriched flour.

Recommended Daily Dietary Allowance (RDA): Infants 10 - 60 micrograms, mcg.; children 20 - 200 mcg.; adults 50 - 200 mcg.

Claimed Benefits Of Taking Supplements: Few, if any, people in the United States suffer obvious deficiency symptoms, because food from selenium-rich areas is widely distributed in the United States. But, people in the United States and in other countries who consume relatively low levels of selenium have much higher rates of heart disease, stroke and cancer than people who live in areas where selenium consumption is relatively high. It is thought that eating foods which are fairly rich in selenium can help prevent some cases of heart disease, stroke and cancer. Using selenium to help prevent these diseases is undergoing medical investigation.

Reported Side Effects And Unsafe Doses: Most medical authorities are concerned that selenium supplementation could be poisonous, because selenium poisoning can occur at intake levels of only a few times the RDA. People who advocate taking selenium supplements caution that supplements should only be used to bring intake levels up to the tops of the RDA figures. Selenium poisoning can cause nausea and loss of hair, fingernails and toenails. Large overdoses can cause death.

Sodium (Sodium Chloride, Salt)

What It Does: Maintains fluid levels between the cells and the blood system . . . acts as an electrolyte to help chemical and electrical reactions in the body.

Food Sources: Sodium is widely distributed in foods and water. It is added to many processed foods and in cooking. The highest natural sources of sodium are dairy products, meat, carrots, poultry, and seafood.

How Long It Stays In The Body: The body conserves sodium by passing very little through the kidneys into the urine when the amount of sodium in the body is low. To a lesser extent, the body also conserves sodium when perspiring. Chloride is usually in balance with sodium, but after excessive vomiting, excessive chloride may be lost. Chloride which is lost in vomiting should be replaced intravenously to avoid hypochloremic metabolic alkalosis.

Deficiency Diseases And Symptoms: Sodium deficiency is almost unknown. Symptoms of sodium deficiency may include weight loss, arthritis, nerve pain, and muscle shrinkage. A severe deficiency of sodium chloride could cause dehydration and death.

What Reduces, Destroys Or Increases It: Diuretic drugs are the chief offenders in throwing off excessive sodium from the body. Excessive sweating can reduce sodium in the body to low levels.

Recommended Daily Dietary Allowance (RDA): Infants 115 - 750 mg.; children 325 - 1800 mg.; adolescents 900 - 2700 mg.; adults 1100 - 3300 mg. **Note:** The recommended daily allowances for sodium may be high, especially for adolescents and adults. In most cases, people should strive to maintain their sodium intake at the lower levels of the ranges. Pregnant or nursing women, or people who sweat a lot because of hard work or exercise, usually should not try to restrict sodium intake drastically.

Claimed Benefits Of Taking Supplements: Pregnant women often can avoid toxemia or pre-eclampsia late in pregnancy by taking adequate sodium, calcium and magnesium and by maintaining good nutritional habits.

Most people in the United States would receive a substantial health benefit by reducing the amount of sodium in the diet instead of supplementing sodium.

Reported Side Effects And Unsafe Doses: Medically supervised, low-sodium diets are often recommended for good health. They seem to reduce the chances of high blood pressure and associated heart and blood vessel disorders in some people. Some doctors prescribe low-sodium diets in which the intake of sodium may be about one-half the lower end of the RDA range. Many adults can maintain adequate sodium in the body with intake at 500 mg. per day unless they sweat a lot or take certain prescription drugs such as diuretics. Some people who have problems with high blood pressure may find substantial relief by restricting their sodium intake to rather low levels.

Excessive sodium in the diet contributes to hypertension or high blood pressure in many people who are salt-sensitive. Sodium chloride can be fatal in adults in doses of approximately one tablespoon. A person could consume this much after drinking seawater. Fortunately, most people will vomit when they consume this much. Eating high amounts of salt can cause insomnia or loss of sleep.

Zinc

What It Does: Involved in many enzyme systems . . . involved in the synthesis of nucleic acid (DNA & RNA), so it is directly related to growth and repair of the body . . . helps burns and wounds heal . . . helps B vitamins work . . . helps in the digestion of carbohydrates and in the proper functioning of the reproduction system . . . helps immune system function and protects against air pollution.

Food Sources: Liver, seafood, dairy products, meat and eggs are good sources of zinc. Vegetable products are poor sources of zinc. Whole wheat and other whole-grain products contain zinc in a less available form than animal products. There is very little zinc in most water supplies.

How Long It Stays In The Body: Deficiency symptoms show up very soon after the removal of zinc from the diet. Some zinc is stored in the bones, but it is not released in sufficient quantities to prevent deficiency symptoms.

Deficiency Diseases And Symptoms: Loss of appetite, failure to grow, poor skin color and appearance, white spots on the fingernails, slow wound healing, infertility, poor resistance to infections, diabetes, loss of taste, poor night vision, birth defects and behavioral disturbances in the offspring of pregnant women, failure of the testes or ovaries to develop and dwarfism are all possible symptoms of zinc deficiency.

Certain conditions which lower blood zinc levels are chronic diarrhea, cirrhosis of the liver, kidney disease, and diabetes. People with these conditions are unusually prone to zinc deficiency. The elderly may also be unusually prone to zinc deficiency because of changes in their diets. Zinc deficiencies in the elderly may make them more prone to disease.

What Reduces, Destroys Or Increases It: Dietary fiber and dietary phytate found in grains interfere with the absorption of zinc, so people on vegetarian diets may not get adequate supplies. Alcohol and calcium can interfere with the absorption of zinc. Low levels of phosphorus in the diet can interfere with the activity of zinc. The need for zinc is increased in pregnancy, chronic diarrhea, infection and sickle cell anemia. Vitamin D increases the absorption of zinc.

Recommended Daily Dietary Allowance (RDA): Infants 3 - 5 mg.; children 10 mg.; adult males 15 mg.; adult females 15 mg.; pregnant women 20 mg.; nursing mothers 25 mg.

Claimed Benefits Of Taking Supplements: Zinc may reduce: hearing loss from nerve damage, ringing in the ears, enlargement and inflammation of the prostate gland and rates of hair loss in the elderly. Other claimed benefits are: firming up of fragile nails that peel, split, break or are abnormally soft, improvement in psoriasis, acne, infertility and impotence, better appetite, higher rates of growth in children, rapid wound healing, improved sense of taste and lower rates of alcoholism and heart disease.

Anorexia nervosa, a serious loss of appetite, has been successfully treated with zinc supplements in 80% of patients in a controlled scientific study. However, professional counseling may help find the cause that triggered the disorder.

Zinc lozenges given every other waking hour have been

reported to speed recovery times in people with the common cold. Zinc supplements taken by mouth and swallowed instead of sucked are reported not to have any benefit in curing colds.

Reported Side Effects And Unsafe Doses: People taking levels close to the RDA usually experience few side effects, but higher doses of 10 times the RDA or more can produce liver disease with lethargy, pain in the stomach and fever. Doses of 7 times the RDA may cause undesirable changes in blood chemistry, particularly lowering beneficial HDL cholesterol. High doses of zinc can drive out other metals from the body and cause anemia. Overdoses of zinc can cause nausea, anemia, stomach pain, premature birth and stillbirth. Doses of 2 grams of zinc sulfate will cause vomiting, and zinc sulfate is sometimes used as an emetic.

One side effect of zinc supplementation is increased appetite and increased weight gain. Children who took zinc supplements in one study consumed 600 more calories per day than children who did not take supplements. The children who took zinc supplements also grew a quarter inch per year more than children who did not take supplements.

A Key Amino Acid

Lysine

What It Does: Lysine is an amino acid. Amino acids are the building blocks which form protein, which is essential for the body to use in its repair and growth. Lysine is considered to be a key amino acid, because it is often deficient in low-protein diets.

Food Sources: Dairy products are the richest source of lysine. Lysine is also found in high concentrations in seafood and meat. Foods which are low in lysine are peanuts, peanut butter and other nut products.

How Long It Stays In The Body: The body can use its own lysine for essential repair and maintenance, but lysine deficiency in the diet will eventually contribute to loss of muscle and malnutrition.

Deficiency Diseases And Symptoms: Poor growth and malnutrition.

What Reduces, Destroys Or Increases It: The amino acid arginine, which is found in high concentrations in peanuts and nut products, counteracts some of the benefits claimed for lysine.

Recommended Daily Dietary Allowance (RDA):
Infants 396 - 891 mg.; children 440 - 1760 mg.; adults
480 - 900 mg.

Claimed Benefits Of Taking Supplements: New
studies suggest that high levels of lysine in the diet,
when combined with low levels of arginine, can give the
body increased resistance to viruses, particularly the
herpes simplex virus. A number of studies now in
progress indicate that the recurrence of herpes infections
can be greatly reduced by a high lysine, low arginine diet
or by taking lysine supplements while avoiding nuts and
other foods which are high in arginine.

There are also studies underway which indicate that high
amounts of lysine in the diet may be an important factor
in preventing some types of cancer.

Reported Side Effects And Unsafe Doses: Diets high
in protein can contribute to osteoporosis and heart
disease. Supplementation by eating foods which are
high in lysine should be balanced against the possible
side effects of consuming large quantities of meat or
dairy products.

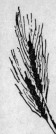

Other Books to Consult

The following is a sample of a large number of book titles which are available on the subject of Vitamins (descriptions of titles are from the publishers).

The Book Of Vitamin Therapy. A doctor tells what megavitamins can do for you. (By Dr. Harold Rosenberg; G P. Putnam's Sons, New York) 1980.

Cancer and Vitamin C. A discussion of the nature, causes, prevention and treatment of cancer. (By Ewan Cameron and Linus Pauling, Ph.D.; Linus Pauling Institute of Science and Medicine, Menlo Park, Ca.) 1979.

The Complete Book of Vitamins, All-New Edition. A one-volume nutritional library of health and healing with vitamins. (By the Staff of Prevention® Magazine; Rodale Press, Emmaus, Pa.) 1984.

The Essential Guide To Nonprescription Drugs. Facts you should know about nonprescription drugs. (David R. Zimmerman; Harper & Row, New York) 1983

Life Extension. A practical scientific approach for adding years to your life and life to your years. (By Durk Pearson and Sandy Shaw; Warner Books, Inc., New York) 1982.

Drug Facts And Comparisons. Drug information for health care professionals. (Facts and Comparisons Division, J. B. Lippincott Company, St. Louis, Missouri) 1984.

Fluoride: The Aging Factor. An account of how fluoride damages the body's repair and rejuvenation capabilities. (By John Yiamouyiannis; Health Action Press, Delaware, Ohio) 1983.

Megavitamin Therapy. Great breakthrough for drug addicts, alcoholics, and the mentally ill. (By Ruth Adams and Frank Murray; Larchmont Books, New York) 1974.

Nutritive Value of Foods. Table of nutritive values for household measures of commonly used foods. (United States Department of Agriculture, prepared by Science and Education Administration, Washington, D. C.) 1981.

Physician's Desk Reference (also referred to as **PDR**). Prescription drug guide published annually with the cooperation of the drug manufacturers. (Medical Economics Company, Oradell, New Jersey) 1984.

The Physician's and Pharmacist's Guide To Your Medicines. The most comprehensive advice for the patient. (By the US Pharmacopeial Convention; Ballantine Books, New York) 1980.

The Pritikin Promise: 28 Days To A Longer, Healthier Life. (By Nathan Pritikin; Simon and Schuster, New York) 1983.

Psychodietetics. Food as the key to emotional health. (By E. Cheraskin, M. D., D.M.D. and W. M. Ringsdorf, Jr., D.M.D.,M.S. Bantam Books, New York) 1974.

Recommended Dietary Allowances. A study supported by The National Institutes of Health and the U.S. Public Health Service. (Office of Publications, National Academy of Sciences, Washington, D. C.) 1980.

Selenium As Food & Medicine. Important, up-to-date information and research on the remarkable mineral that protects you. (By Dr. Richard A. Passwater; Keats Publishing, New Canaan, Connecticut) 1980.

Vitamin Bible. A nutritionist/pharmacist gives you all the facts about vitamins. (By Earl Mindell; Warner Books, New York) 1981.

The Vitamin Book. A complete guide to vitamins, minerals and essential nutrients. (By Rich Wentzler; Gramercy Publishing Company, New York) 1980.

The Vitamin C Connection. Scientific research that connects vitamin C to the prevention and treatment of many common health problems. (Dr. E. Cheraskin, Dr. W. M. Ringsdorf, Jr. and Dr. Emily Sisley; Harper and Row, New York) 1983.

Vitamin C and the Common Cold. How to avoid colds and improve your health. (Linus Pauling, Ph. D.; W. H. Freeman and Company, San Francisco, Ca.) 1970.

Vitamin C, the Common Cold, and the Flu. This book changed the nutritional habits of millions. (By Linus Pauling, Ph.D.; W. H. Freeman and Company, San Francisco, Ca.) 1976.

Vitamin C, The Protective Vitamin. The latest facts about the extraordinary health vitamin. (By James Webster; Universal-Award House, Inc., New York) 1971.

Vitamin E Your Key To A Healthy Heart. The suppressed record of the curative values of this remarkable vitamin. (By Herbert Bailey; ARC Books, Inc. New York) 1971.

The Vitamin Pioneers. All about vitamins...What they are...How they were discovered...How they keep us healthy. (By Herbert Bailey; Pyramid Publications, New York, N. Y.) 1970.

Vitamins & You. Tells you what to buy and when to take it. (By Robert J. Benowicz; Berkley Publishing Group, New York) 1983.

Which Vitamins Do You Need? Handbook with everything you need to know about all 17 vitamins. (By Martin Ebon; Bantam Books, New York) 1976.

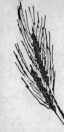

Index: Including How To Locate Vitamins or Minerals Which May Help or Cause Certain Conditions

abdominal discomfort . . . . . . .thiamine (B1), calcium
Accutane® . . . . A
acetaminophen . . . . B12, folic acid
acne . . . . A, pyridoxine (B6), zinc
adaptation to cold . . . . .magnesium
adrenal glands . . . . .pantothenic acid (B5),
                             pyridoxine (B6), C, E
aging, *rapid* . . . . fluoride, selenium
        reduced rate of . . . . . . E
alcohol, *alcoholism* . . . . A, thiamine (B1), riboflavin
                             (B2), niacin (B3), pantothenic
                             acid (B5) pyridoxine (B6),
                             C, biotin, folic acid, calcium
                             magnesium, zinc
Alzheimer's disease . . . . choline
amphetamines C
anemia . . . . .riboflavin (B2), pyridoxine
                             (B6), folic acid, copper
anemia, *hemolytic* . . . . E, iron
anemia, *pernicious* . . . . B12, folic acid
anorexia nervosa . . . . .zinc
Antabuse® C
antacid preparations . . . . niacin (B3), D
antibiotics . . . . thiamine (B1), riboflavin (B2),
                             niacin (B3), biotin, inositol

anticoagulants . . . . pantothenic acid (B5), C, E, K
anticonvulsant . . . . .D
antidepressants C
antihypertensive drugs . . . . . pantothenic acid (B5)
anxiety . . . . inositol
appearance . . . . zinc
appetite . . . . niacin (B3), thiamine (B1),
                                    pantothenic acid (B5), B12,
                                    biotin, folic acid, calcium,
                                    phosphorus, zinc
arteries, *damage* . . . . calcium, pyridoxine (B6),
                                    copper
         hardening of . . . . . . calcium, pyridoxine (B6), C, E
arthritis . . . . .pantothenic acid (B5)
                                    pyridoxine (B6), C, sodium
asthma . . . . .A, pyridoxine (B6)
                                    manganese, C
aspirin . . . . .C, K, folic acid
bad breath . . . . .niacin (B3)
baking soda . . . . riboflavin (B2)
balance . . . . pantothenic (B5), D
baldness, *prevention of* . . . . . .thiamine (B2), inositol
barbiturate . . . . .pyridoxine (B6), D
bed rest, prolonged . . . . .calcium
behavioral disturbances . . . . .zinc
Bendectin® . . . . .pyridoxine (B6)
beri-beri . . . . thiamine (B1)
bioflavonoids C
birth control pills . . . . *see oral contraceptives*
birth defects . . . . riboflavin (B2), pyridoxine
                                    (B6), folic acid, manganese,
                                    zinc
birth, *premature* . . . . zinc
birth weight . . . . fluoride
bladder cancer . . . . inositol
bleeding . . . . .K
blood cell abnormality . . . . . .copper

blood clots . . . . .E, calcium, magnesium
blood disorders . . . . pyridoxine (B6)
blood loss . . . . iron
blood pressure . . . . niacin (B3), pantothenic acid
                                  (B5), D, E, calcium, choline
                                  iron, potassium, sodium
blood sugar levels . . . . niacin (B3), pantothenic acid
                                  (B5), C, chromium,
                                  manganese
blood vessel disorders . . . . . C, D, sodium
bones, *cracks* . . . . D, fluoride
      deformities. . . . . D
      disease . . . . .copper
      formation . . . . .calcium, manganese,
                        phosphorus
      health of . . . . .D, calcium, copper,
                        phosphorus
      knots . . . . fluoride
      marrow . . . . biotin
      pain . . . . fluoride, D, phosphorus,
                        calcium
      strength . . . . fluoride
bowel movements, *excessive* magnesium
bow legs . . . . D
brain, *covering* B12
      function C
breast enlargement . . . . E
breathing difficulty . . . . iron
bruising . . . . .C, K
bruxism . . . . .pantothenic acid (B5)
burning sensations . . . . .thiamine (B1), pantothenic acid
                                  (B5)
caffeine . . . . pantothenic acid (B5),
                                  pyridoxine (B6), calcium
                                  iron, inositol
calcium propionate B12
cancer . . . . A, C, chromium, fluoride,

carpal tunnel syndrome . . . . . pyridoxine (B6)
cartilage . . . . .manganese
cataracts . . . . riboflavin (B2), niacin (B3)
cavities . . . . .fluoride
chest pain . . . . .thiamine (B1)
chills . . . . .D
chloramphenicol B12
chlorine . . . . E
cholesterol levels . . . . .C, inositol
cholestyramine . . . . .D
                                     selenium, lysine, inositol
carbohydrate metabolism . . . niacin (B3), thiamine (B1),
                                     chromium, magnesium,
                                     manganese, zinc
cigarettes . . . . *see smoking*
circulation . . . . niacin (B3), E, chromium
cirrhosis . . . . .inositol, zinc
claudication, *intermittent* . . . . E
clotting . . . . K, calcium
cocaine C
codeine B12
coffee . . . . niacin (B3), iron,
                                     see also caffeine
colitis . . . . iron
collagen formation C
common cold . . . . A, C, zinc
concentration . . . . .thiamine (B1)
confusion . . . . B12, folic acid, magnesium
congestion . . . . D
conjunctivitis . . . . .A
constipation . . . . .thiamine (B1), pantothenic acid
                                     (B5), C, D, calcium, inositol,
                                     iron, magnesium, potassium
convulsions . . . . .pyridoxine (B6), magnesium
co-ordination . . . . .manganese
coronary heart disease . . . . . . pyridoxine (B6), magnesium
cortisone . . . . .D, pyridoxine (B6), calcium

Coumadin® . . . . K
cramps . . . . .thiamine (B1), pantothenic acid
(B5), D, E, calcium,
magnesium
crystals in the kidneys C
deformities, *bone* . . . .*see bone*
dehydration . . . . A, sodium
depression . . . . thiamine (B1), riboflavin (B2),
niacin (B3), pantothenic acid
(B5), pyridoxine (B6), B12, C,
biotin, folic acid, iron
magnesium
development . . . . D, iodine
diabetes, *mellitus* . . . . chromium, thiamine (B1), C,
folic acid, manganese, zinc
see also blood sugar levels
dialysis . . . . fluoride
diarrhea . . . . .thiamine (B1), niacin (B3),
pantothenic acid (B5), B12,C, D,
choline, folic acid, magnesium,
zinc
Dicumarol® . . . . .K
digestive system *deterioration* A
disorders . . . niacin (B3)
function of . . pantothenic acid (B5)
digitalis . . . . C, D
Dilantin® . . . . pyridoxine (B6), folic acid
disulfiram C
diuretics . . . . .magnesium
diuretics, *thiazide* . . . . D, potassium, sodium
dizziness . . . . .thiamine (B1), niacin (B3),
pantothenic acid (B5),
choline, manganese
dolomite . . . . .calcium, niacin (B3)
dryness of mouth . . . . .calcium
dwarfism . . . . zinc
dysplasia of the cervix . . . . . . folic acid

ears, *ringing in the*.......... D, choline, manganese, zinc
eclampsia.................. pyridoxine (B6), sodium
eczema................... inositol
edema.................... pyridoxine (B6), *see also*
                              fluid retention
emetic.................... zinc
emotional stress........... *see stress*
emphysema................ A
energy, *lack of*............ biotin
        increased.......... pyridoxine (B6)
epilepsy.................. folic acid
estradiol................. folic acid
estrogens................. thiamine (B1), pyridoxine (B6)
excitability............... niacin (B3), magnesium
exercise.................. thiamine (B1), riboflavin
                              (B2), niacin (B3), calcium
exostoses................. fluoride
eyelids, *inflamed*.......... riboflavin (B2)
        thickened.......... A
eyes, *bloodshot*............ riboflavin (B2)
     burning.............. A
     disintegration of eyeball A
     health of............ E, inositol
     itching................ A
     lining of............ riboflavin (B2)
     sore.................. D
eye whites, *cloudy*........... A
fainting.................. niacin (B3)
fat, *breaking down of*........ inositol
fat levels.................. C
fatigue................... thiamine (B1), riboflavin (B2),
                              niacin (B3), pantothenic acid (B5),
                              pyridoxine (B6), B12, C, E, folic
                              acid, iron, inositol, manganese
fertility.................. B12, C, choline, manganese,
                              zinc
fever.................... C, zinc

fibrocystic breast disease ...	E	
fingernails,	*health of*	riboflavin (B2), iron, zinc
	loss of	selenium
	white spots	zinc
fluid levels	sodium	
fluid retention	thiamine (B1), pyridoxine (B6), C, potassium	
fontanels, *bulging*	A	
gallbladder, *function of*	choline	
genital areas	A	
glaucoma	A, niacin (B3), D, choline	
goiter	iodine	
gout	niacin (B3)	
growth	A, thiamine (B1), pyridoxine (B6), B12, C, D, calcium, fluoride, lysine, manganese, phosphorus, zinc	
gums,	*health of*	C
hair,	*brittle*	A
	dry	A, C, iodine
	formation of	copper
	health of	riboflavin (B2), biotin, inositol
	loss of	A, pyridoxine (B6), biotin, inositol, selenium, zinc
	pigmentation of	copper
	structure of	copper
hallucinations	niacin (B3)	
hardening of the arteries ...	pyridoxine (B6)	
headaches	niacin (B3), C, E, iron	
healing	C, copper, zinc	
hearing,	*loss of*	fluoride, zinc
	problems	manganese
heart,	*attack*	potassium
	coronary heart disease.	pyridoxine (B6), magnesium
	damage	copper
	disease	C, E, folic acid, potassium,

selenium, zinc
disorders . . . . sodium, selenium
failure . . . . D
irregular beat . . . . niacin (B3), C, D, potassium
pain . . . . B12, biotin, folic acid
palpitations . . . . iodine
poor function . . . . E, thiamine (B1), chromium
poor rhythm . . . . A
proper function . . . . . . calcium, inositol, magnesium
pounding heartbeat . . . B12, folic acid, calcium
skipped beats . . . . niacin (B3)
heartburn . . . . niacin (B3)
hemoglobin formation . . . . . . C, copper, iron
hemolytic anemia . . . . *see anemia*
hemorrhoids . . . . iron
herpes simplex virus . . . . lysine
high blood pressure . . . . niacin (B3), D, E, choline,
calcium, potassium, sodium
high blood sugar . . . . chromium, manganese
homocystinuria . . . . pyridoxine (B6)
hormone regulation . . . . riboflavin (B2), niacin (B3),
pantothenic acid (B5), manganese
hot flashes . . . . E
hot weather . . . . calcium, fluoride
hunchback . . . . fluoride
hydralazine . . . . pyridoxine (B6)
hyperglycemia . . . . chromium
hypertension . . . . *see high blood pressure*
hyperthyroidism . . . . A, riboflavin (B2)
hypocalcemia . . . . D
hypochloremic metabolic
  alkalosis . . . . sodium
hypoglycemia . . . . niacin (B3), chromium
hypothyroidism . . . . iodine
ileitis B12
ileus . . . . pantothenic acid (B5)
immune system
  development . . . . C, E, choline, zinc

immunological disorders . . . . riboflavin (B2), choline
impotence . . . . zinc
indigestion . . . . .pantothenic acid (B5), C, E
infections . . . . A, pantothenic acid (B5), C, E,
                                               iron, chromium, zinc
infertility . . . . zinc, *see also fertility*
insomnia . . . . thiamine (B1), niacin (B3),
                                               pyridoxine (B6), D, calcium,
                                               iron, potassium, sodium
insulin . . . . pyridoxine (B6), chromium
intelligence . . . . thiamine (B1)
interferon C
intermittent claudication . . . .E
intestinal tract . . . . .folic acid
intestines . . . . A, thiamine (B1)
    bleeding . . . . iron
    discomfort . . . . C, D
    distress . . . . E
intrauterine devices (IUD) . . . . iron
irritability . . . . A, thiamine (B1), niacin
                                               (B3), iron, iodine, magnesium,
                                             potassium
isoniazid . . . . .pyridoxine (B6)
itching . . . . A, niacin (B3), D
jaundice . . . . .E, K
kidneys . . . . .C, D, choline, inositol
    calcium deposits . . . . . . .D
    damage . . . . .choline
    dialysis machines . . . . . .fluoride
    disease . . . . zinc
    problems . . . . .potassium
kidney stones . . . . .pyridoxine (B6), C, calcium,
                                               magnesium
knock knees . . . . .D
laxatives . . . . .D, K
learning . . . . pyridoxine (B6), thiamine (B1)
lecithin . . . . .choline

lethargy . . . . zinc
levodopa . . . . pyridoxine (B6)
lightheadedness . . . . D
light sensitivity . . . . riboflavin (B2), D
lips, *cracked* . . . . A, pyridoxine (B6)
      irritated . . . . pyridoxine (B6)
      pale or red . . . . riboflavin (B2)
      sore . . . . pyridoxine (B6)
liver . . . . thiamine (B1), niacin (B3),
                                            D, K, biotin, choline,
                                            inositol, selenium, zinc
loss of feeling . . . . thiamine (B1)
loss of hair . . . . *see hair*
loss of hearing . . . . *see hearing*
loss of position . . . . pyridoxine (B6)
loss of reflexes . . . . pyridoxine (B6), B12
loss of sensation . . . . pyridoxine (B6)
low blood pressure . . . . niacin (B3), pantothenic acid (B5)
low blood sugar . . . . pantothenic acid (B5), chromium
                                            see also blood sugar levels
lung deterioration . . . . A
lungs . . . . A, D, E
malnutrition . . . . lysine
margarine . . . . E
marijuana C
marrow, bone . . . . biotin
maturity-onset diabetes . . . . . chromium
measles . . . . A
memory . . . . thiamine (B1), choline
menopausal arthritis . . . . pyridoxine (B6)
menopause . . . . calcium, E
mental attitude . . . . thiamine (B1), iodine
mental confusion . . . . thiamine (B1)
mental illness . . . . choline, D, niacin
mental retardation . . . . pyridoxine (B6), iodine
metabolism . . . . E, phosphorus
methotrexate . . . . folic acid

methylbromide . . . . pantothenic acid (B5)
migraines . . . . A, *see also headaches*
mineral metabolism . . . . .magnesium
miscarriages . . . . .manganese
molybdenum . . . . copper
mood changes . . . . .pantothenic acid (B5)
morning sickness . . . . pyridoxine (B6)
motion sickness . . . . .pyridoxine (B6)
mouth,   *dry* . . . . .calcium
            health of . . . . A
            numbness . . . . pyridoxine (B6)
            pain . . . . .riboflavin (B2)
            sore . . . . .niacin (B3), pyridoxine (B6),
                                         B12, folic acid, iron
mucous membranes
            genital areas . . . . A
            intestines . . . . A
            lungs. . . . . .A
            mouth . . . . .A, pyridoxine (B6)
            pain of . . . . riboflavin (B2)
            stomach . . . . A
            throat . . . . .A
muscle,   *contractions* . . . . . . calcium, magnesium
            co-ordination . . . . . manganese
            cramps . . . . E, pantothenic acid (B5), calcium
            deterioration . . . . . .E, lysine, selenium
            function . . . . .calcium, inositol, E, phosphorus,
                                         potassium
            formation . . . . E
            incoordination . . . . .manganese
            pain . . . . .biotin
            shrinkage . . . . .sodium
            spasms . . . . .D
            tone . . . . .thiamine (B1), D, inositol
            tremors . . . . A, magnesium
            uncontrollable
                movements . . B12, choline

weakness . . . . niacin (B3)
muscular dystrophy . . . . .inositol
nails, *health of* . . . . .riboflavin (B2), iron, zinc
nausea .thiamine (B1), riboflavin (B2),
niacin (B3), pantothenic acid
(B5),biotin, calcium, selenium,
zinc
necrotising enterocolitis . . . . . E
neomycin B12
nerve cell development . . . . . . folic acid
nerves, *damage* . . . . .zinc
    function of . . . . biotin, phosphorus
    pain . . . . sodium
    transmission of impulses. thiamine (B1)
nervousness . . . . riboflavin (B2), niacin (B3),
pyridoxine (B5), D, iodine,
magnesium
nervous system,
    degeneration . . . . copper
    deterioration B12
    disorders . . . . niacin (B3)
    function . . . . calcium, inositol
    maintenance . . . . folic acid, potassium
neutropenia . . . . copper
nicotine . . . . .pyridoxine (B6)
night vision . . . . A
numbness . . . . pyridoxine (B6), B12
nursing mothers . . . . calcium, sodium
obesity . . . . iodine
oil glands . . . . biotin
oral contraceptives . . . . A, thiamine (B1), riboflavin (B2),
niacin (B3), pyridoxine (B6),
B12, C, E, copper, folic acid,
calcium, iron, K
osteoarthritis . . . . pantothenic acid (B5)
osteomalacia . . . . D, calcium, fluoride
osteoporosis . . . . calcium, choline, fluoride,
phosphorus

otospongeosis . . . . fluoride
ovaries . . . . biotin, zinc
oxygen therapy . . . . E
pain . . . . riboflavin (B2), pantothenic
                                            acid (B5), pyridoxine (B6), C, D,
                                            see also location of pain
pancreas inflammation . . . . . . D
paralysis . . . . thiamine (B1), B12, biotin
paralytic ileus . . . . pantothenic acid (B5)
parathyroid function . . . . calcium
pellagra . . . . niacin (B3)
penicillamine . . . . pyridoxine (B6)
peptic ulcers . . . . iron
pernicious anemia . . . . B12, folic acid
phenobarbital . . . . folic acid
phenytoin . . . . pyridoxine (B6)
pollution . . . . E, zinc
position, *loss of* . . . . pyridoxine (B6)
pregnancy . . . . K, calcium, sodium, zinc
premature birth . . . . E, zinc
pre-menstrual acne . . . . pyridoxine (B6)
pre-menstrual fluid
        retention . . . . pyridoxine (B6)
pre-menstrual weight gain . . pyridoxine (B6)
pressure within the skull . . . . A
primidone . . . . folic acid
prostate gland . . . . zinc
protein metabolism . . . . niacin (B3), manganese
prothrombin production . . . . K
psoriasis . . . . zinc
psychoses . . . . pantothenic acid (B5), B12
pulmonary embolism . . . . E
pyrimethamine . . . . folic acid
rash . . . . niacin (B3), folic acid
red blood cell production . . . . pyridoxine (B6), C, E,
                                            copper, folic acid, iron
reflexes . . . . thiamine (B1), pyridoxine (B6),
                                            B12, potassium

repair of body . . . . lysine, zinc
reproduction . . . . manganese, zinc
reproductive organ damage. . E
reproductive system . . . . A, copper
resistance . . . . iron, lysine
respiratory infection . . . . pantothenic acid (B5)
respiratory,
      shortness of breath . . . . B12, folic acid
restlessness . . . . D
retinopathy . . . . E
Reye's syndrome C
rheumatoid arthritis . . . . pantothenic acid (B5)
rickets . . . . D, calcium
ringing in the ears . . . . D, manganese, zinc
runners . . . . E, iron
saccharin . . . . biotin
schizophrenia . . . . niacin (B3), C
scleroderma . . . . fluoride
scurvy C
senility . . . . pantothenic acid (B5)
sensitivity to light . . . . riboflavin (B2), D
sex drive, *decreased* . . . . D
sex hormone production . . . . C, manganese
sex organs . . . . folic acid
sexual function, *reduction of* . E
shortening . . . . E
shortness of breath . . . . B12, folic acid
sickle cell anemia . . . . zinc
skin,   *bleeding under* C
      blemished . . . . A
      cracked . . . . A
      dermatitis . . . . niacin (B3)
      diseases . . . . biotin
      dry . . . . A, niacin (B3), C, biotin, iodine
      flushed . . . . niacin (B3)
      formation . . . . copper
      functions of . . . . A, biotin
      greasy .   . . . riboflavin (B2)

hard patches	fluoride
health of	A, riboflavin (B2), niacin (B3), inositol
inflexible	niacin (B3)
pale	iron
peeling	A
poor color	zinc
rash.	niacin (B3), folic acid
red	riboflavin (B2), niacin (B3), biotin
smoothness	A
scaly	riboflavin (B2), niacin (B3), biotin
sores	niacin (B3), C
wrinkling	pantothenic acid (B5), E, fluoride
yellow	E

skull, *pressure* .... A
     soft spots .... A
sleep disturbances . ... *see insomnia*
sleeping pills .... niacin (B3)
sleeplessness .... biotin, choline, *see also insomnia*
smell, *sense of* .... A
smoking .... A, thiamine (B1), C, D, calcium
soreness of mouth, *tongue* .... B12, folic acid
stamina .... pantothenic acid (B5), iron
sterility .... E
steroids .... pantothenic acid (B5)
stiffness .... fluoride
stillbirth .... zinc
stomach, *acidity* .... magnesium
     bleeding .... niacin (B3), iron
     calcium deposits .. D
     cancer C
     discomfort .... C, D

movement	thiamine (B1)
mucous membranes.	A
nausea	*see nausea*
pain	zinc
ulcers	niacin (B3), C, choline
upset	*see nausea*
stress	thiamine (B1), niacin (B3), pantothenic acid (B5), pyridoxine (B6), C, calcium, iron, magnesium
stroke	selenium
sulfa drugs	thiamine (B1), niacin (B3), C, biotin, folic acid
sunburn	C
surgery	C
sweat glands	biotin
swelling	thiamine (B1), E
tardive dyskinesia	niacin (B3), choline
Tartrazine®	niacin (B3)
taste, *loss of*	zinc
teeth, *brown*	fluoride
decay	calcium, pyridoxine (B6)
enamel	A, fluoride
formation	D, phosphorus
grinding	pantothenic acid (B5)
loss of	C
pitted	fluoride
white	fluoride
temperature, *sense of*	pyridoxine (B6)
testes	biotin, zinc
testosterone	folic acid
tetany	calcium
tetracycline	calcium, iron
thiazide diuretics	D
thirst	D, calcium, potassium
Thorazine®	niacin (B3)
throat	A
thyroid function	E

thyroid gland enlargement . . . .iodine
thyroid hormones . . . . .choline
tingling sensation B12
tiredness . . . . *see fatigue*
tissue formation . . . . A, thiamine (B1), riboflavin
                           (B2), E
tobacco . . . . *see smoking*
toenails . . . . selenium
tongue, *purplish* . . . . riboflavin (B2)
       red . . . . .niacin (B3)
       sore . . . . riboflavin (B2), niacin (B3),
                            B12, folic acid
                            niacin (B3)
     swollen . . . . pyridoxine (B6)
touch, *sense of* . . . . .pyridoxine (B6), sodium
toxemia . . . . folic acid
triamterene C
tricyclic antidepressants . . . . . niacin (B3), pyridoxine (B6)
tryptophan . . . . .choline, *see also cancer*
tumors . . . . *see acetaminophen*
Tylenol® . . . . riboflavin (B2), niacin (B3),
ulcers . . . . pyridoxine (B6), C

unsteady walking . . . . .pantothenic acid (B5), B12
upset stomach . . . . *see nausea*
urinary system deterioration . A
urinary tract stone formation.C
urination, *increased* . . . . .D, calcium
        painful . . . . .D
vegetable oils . . . . E
verapamil . . . . .D, calcium
vibration sense, *loss of* . . . . . . pyridoxine (B6)
viral meningitis C
vision . . . . .A, riboflavin (B2), pyridoxine
                            (B6), choline, zinc
vomiting . . . . A, niacin (B3), C, D, biotin,
                            calcium, zinc
weakness . . . . pantothenic acid (B5), fluoride,

	phosphorus, potassium
weight gain	B12, pyridoxine (B6), zinc
weight loss	thiamine (B1)
white blood cells	E, folic acid
wounds, *healing of*	C, zinc

"HE DIED WITH ARTERIES LIKE A BABY"

Clean Artery

Artery 50% clogged by fat and cholesterol

Artery 90% clogged by fat and cholesterol

(By Frank K. Wood)

Can your arteries be cleaned out naturally? That's what many doctors are wondering after an autopsy of a famous nutrition expert.

The "free from artery disease" theory of the nutrition expert may be proven by his death! The doctor who performed the autopsy was, in his own words, "amazed to find no evidence of coronary artery disease in a man of his age (69)". He said that the nutrition expert died with "arteries like a baby". What's even more amazing is that the nutrition expert was diagnosed as actually having coronary artery disease 30 years earlier when he was 39 years old.

Case studies like the well-known nutritionist's may be atypical. Now, a new book, *"Arteries Cleaned Out Naturally"* contains information on a natural, drug free way to stop heart and artery disease.

LIFE SAVING SECRETS REVEALED IN THIS NEW BOOK

- How to tell if you're having a heart attack... or just indigestion.
- A new treatment that opens up arteries without surgery.
- Amazing, easy ways to keep your arteries clean.
- A simple step that can help 1/3 of all Americans avoid a heart attack.
- Why foot problems are associated with high rates of heart attack.
- Exercise. . . one type that's very harmful . . . another type that can help.
- Definitions of terms like coronary thrombosis, aneurysm, angina, etc.
- The amazing story of HDL's. The body's natural system that helps keep the arteries clean.
- How to add 10 years to your life.
- The truth about cholesterol and hardening of the arteries.

IT'S EASY TO ORDER

Just return this notice with your name and address and a check for **$11.97** plus $3.00 shipping and handling to our address: **FC&A, Dept. XMZ-2,** 103 Clover Green, Peachtree City, Georgia 30269. We will send you a copy of *"Arteries Cleaned Out Naturally"* right away.

Save! Return this notice with **$23.94** + $3.00 for two books. (No extra shipping and handling charges.)

Satisfaction guaranteed or your money back.

Cut out and return this notice with your order. Copies not accepted!

IMPORTANT — FREE GIFT OFFER

All orders will receive a free gift. Order right away!

©FC&A 1988